## Advance Praise For *THE ESSENTIAL COSMETIC SURGERY COM*

Dr. Kotler has presented yet another gift [...] tic surgery with this step-by-step workbook to [...] on. Every cosmetic surgeon will welcome the patient [...] e it keeps the consultation focused on the important issues.

—Jeremy L. Freeman, MD, FACS, FRCS (C)
Professor, University of Toronto

Dr. Kotler provides the important questions that only a cosmetic surgeon would now to ask. His agenda-like format is what patients – and doctors – need to stay on target during their consultation. Highly recommended.

—Linda Li, MD, FACS
Featured plastic surgeon on E! Entertainment's *Dr. 90210*

Once again, Dr. Kotler it at the forefront of patient education. This unique workbook is the logical sequel to last year's superb primer, **SECRETS OF A BEVERLY HILLS COSMETIC SURGEON**. Advances in cosmetic surgery – while beneficial – make decision-making more difficult. To have a successful result, patient's need guidance and direction. Now, from one of the specialty's best teachers, they have it.

—Keith Wahl, MD, FACS
Clinical Attending, University of California San Diego

In his latest book, Dr. Robert Kotler coaches patients through the cosmetic surgery consultation process. This user-friendly workbook enables patients to maximize their time with doctor they are consulting with. A powerful new tool for consumers.

—Neil Baum, MD
Tulane University Medical School

If you're even THINKING of cosmetic surgery, BUY THIS BOOK. A terrific guide filled with insider tips.

—Bill Fulcher, MD
Board-certified anesthesiologist featured on
E! Entertainment's *Dr. 90210*

This book puts famous cosmetic surgeon Dr. Robert Kotler at your side as you make your decisions about your own plastic surgery. This expert walks you through the specific questions to ask that will determine if a procedure and a doctor is right for you. I am recommending this book to my patients and viewers.

—Mary Ann Malloy, MD
Cardiologist and Lecturer, Northwestern University
Feinberg School of Medicine
Medical Reporter, NBC 5 Chicago

Dr. Kotler has written another practical book to help patients through the complex maze of cosmetic surgery. The practical checklists full of useful discussion points will help patients to focus on the important issues.

—Robert Alan Goldberg, MD
Professor of Ophthalmology and
Chief, Orbital and Ophthalmic Plastic Surgery, UCLA
Executive Secretary, American Society of
Ophthalmic Plastic and Reconstructive Surgery

With millions of elective cosmetic surgeries in the US alone, I'm delighted that someone has written an authoritative guide on the subject. I'm particularly happy that this someone is Dr. Robert Kotler. His passion and experience, combined with his easy to understand writing style makes this book a must-read for anyone considering cosmetic surgery.

—Howard Murad, MD
Assistant Clinical Professor of Dermatology, UCLA
Founder, Murad, Inc.

Cosmetic surgery in the outpatient setting demands the highest trained and most experienced practitioners in all aspects of patient care. Dr. Kotler, a stalwart advocate for the highest quality of patient care, understands this concept and delivers an important section on outpatient/office-based anesthesia for cosmetic surgery.

—Adam Frederic Dorin, MD, MBA
Board-certified anesthesiologist
Former President, American Society of Anesthesiologists
Editorial Board, Outpatient Surgery Magazine

In our joint interest in maintaining safety through appropriate standards, equipment and personnel via accreditation programs in surgical facilities, this book properly instructs potential patients to research these critical elements in preparation for any surgical procedure.

—James A. Yates, MD
President, American Association for the Accreditation
of Ambulatory Surgery Facilities

# THE ESSENTIAL
# COSMETIC SURGERY
## COMPANION

## Don't Consult a Cosmetic Surgeon Without This Book!

**Robert Kotler, MD, FACS**

*Knowledge exists to be imparted.*

— Ralph Waldo Emerson (1803–1882)

THE ESSENTIAL COSMETIC SURGERY COMPANION
Robert Kotler, MD, FACS

Published by:
Ernest Mitchell Publishers
P.O. Box 15371
Beverly Hills, CA 90209-1371
Phone: 888-599-3400
Info at www.robertkotlermd.com

*Our books are available at special quantity discounts for bulk purchases for sales promotions, premiums, fund-raising, or educational use. For details write Ernest Mitchell Publishers.*

Printed in the United States of America
10 9 8 7 6 5 4 3 2 1
Library of Congress Control Number: 2005927830
ISBN: 0-9712262-2-9 Softbound

---

## Disclaimer

This book is designed to provide information about the subject matter covered.

It is not the purpose of this book to reprint all the information that is otherwise available to the author and/or publisher, but to complement, amplify and supplement. You are urged to read all available material.

Every effort has been made to make this book as complete and as accurate as possible. However, there may be mistakes both typographical and in content. Therefore, this text should be used only as a general guide.

The purpose of this book is to educate. The author and Ernest Mitchell Publishers shall have neither liability nor responsibility to any person or entity with respect to any loss or damage caused, directly or indirectly by the information contained in this book.

---

Text Design: Carolyn Porter, One-On-One Book Production
Cover Design: Amy King
Cover Photos: John Sanchez

# Dedication

*To my thousands of patients who asked good questions.*
*In essence, they wrote this book.*

*And, to*
*Howard Schultz, creator and producer of Extreme Makeover,*
*a man of unusual imagination and creativity,*
*he brought into the homes of millions*
*the recognition of modern cosmetic surgery's*
*and its allies' abilities to improve lives.*

*And, to*
*Donald Bull, Producer and Director of Dr. 90210,*
*the first to open the windows to both*
*the surgeon's professional and personal lives.*
*Real reality television.*

Author royalties are donated to fund continuing leukemia research in honor of my daughter Lauren, a leukemia survivor and patient advocate.

# Table of Contents

# APPENDICES

# ABOUT THE AUTHOR

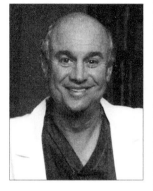 Robert Kotler, MD, FACS, practices cosmetic facial surgery exclusively, in Beverly Hills, California.

Born in Chicago, Dr. Kotler attended the University of Wisconsin and is a graduate of Northwestern University Medical School. He served his general surgery residency at Cook County Hospital in Chicago. His specialty residency training in surgery of the face, head and neck was served at Cook County Hospital, Northwestern University Hospitals, and the University of Illinois Hospitals. Dr. Kotler is board certified by the American Board of Otolaryngology/Head and Neck Surgery.

A former Major, Medical Corps., U.S. Army, Dr. Kotler was Chief of Head and Neck Surgery at the DeWitt Army Hospital, Fort Belvoir, Virginia, and a consultant and residency program instructor at the Walter Reed Army Medical Center, Washington, D.C.

Following his military service, Dr. Kotler served a fellowship in cosmetic facial surgery, sponsored by the American Academy of Facial Plastic and Reconstructive Surgery.

Dr. Kotler is the founder of the Cosmetic Surgery Specialists Medical Group of Beverly Hills. In addition to his private practice, he is a Clinical Instructor in the Division of Head and Neck Surgery, Department of Surgery, UCLA Center for the Health Sciences. He is a Consultant and Attending Surgeon at the Veterans' Medical Center, West Los Angeles. Dr. Kotler has served as a Commissioner and Regional Consultant to the Medical Board of California, and as a Medical Consultant to the City and County of Los Angeles.

Dr. Kotler is the author of *THE CONSUMER'S GUIDEBOOK TO COSMETIC FACIAL SURGERY* and the best-seller, *SECRETS OF A BEVERLY HILLS COSMETIC SURGEON*. He also wrote the medical text, *CHEMICAL REJUVENATION OF THE FACE*, which is used by physicians worldwide. Dr. Kotler is credited with 51 medical publications and presentations, and he has been author or contributor to 14 medical textbooks and books for the public.

As a spokesperson for cosmetic surgeons, Dr. Kotler has been a guest on numerous local and national radio and television programs, including *The Oprah Winfrey Show*, CBS News, *48 Hours*, CNN, Fox News, and he has been interviewed by *Time, Self, McCalls, Men's Health, Allure, Men's Fitness, Los Angeles Magazine, W, Woman's Day, The Chicago Sun-Times, Los Angeles Times, Detroit Press, Arizona Republic, Denver Post, Cincinnati Enquirer, Parade* and *USA Today*.

Dr. Kotler is a featured cosmetic surgeon on E! Entertainment's hit TV series, *Dr. 90210*. His down-to-earth bearing, insightful commentaries, common sense advice and witty humor have endeared him to millions of viewers throughout the world.

# ACKNOWLEDGMENTS

It was a pleasure to reassemble my publishing "kitchen cabinet," those advisors, consultants and friends who were so helpful in the creation of this book's successful ancestor, *SECRETS OF A BEVERLY HILLS COSMETIC SURGEON, The Expert's Guide to Safe, Successful Surgery*.

Our books' distributor, Independent Publishers Group, is a storehouse of solid advice and practical publishing suggestions. Appreciation to Mark Suchomel, Mary Rowles, Mark Voigt, Catherine Bosin, Molly Lyons, Cynthia Murphy and Annie Johnson. These solid Chicagoans were in the boat, rowing with us, all the way.

Jan Nathan and Lisa Krebs of the Publishers Marketing Association always help focus our thinking and cultivate our best work.

Cover designer Amy King, in New York City. Having admired her cover designs for other books, we tracked her down because we wanted her on board for this mission. We were not disappointed.

Cheryl De Poorter faithfully transcribed the manuscript, overcoming the author's "speed-talking" on transcription tapes.

Shannon Melamed managed to successfully punctuate her USC undergrad studies with the in-house editing of the manuscript. Eagle-eyed copy editing by Margery Schwartz.

Appreciation to my loyal and dedicated office staff: Mary Jakubowitz, Agnes Bjelke and Leeza Yaroshevsky, who keep the practice running in high gear as well as supporting my writing efforts.

Irwin Zucker, founder and spiritual leader of the Book Publicists of Southern California; Dr. Earl Mindell, author of 52 books on nutrition; and Melvin Powers, publishing legend and powerhouse. All are willing fountains of wisdom and good advice for any author seeking their counsel. Once again, I did.

My practice associates in the Cosmetic Surgery Specialists Medical Group of Beverly Hills: Les Bolton, MD, FACS, and Athleo "Tel" Cambre, MD, FACS, for their review and input on the body procedures section.

Attorney Stan Coleman and his charming, beautiful and dutiful assistant, Bo Horne. Thanks for dotting the Is and crossing the Ts.

Unending admiration for advisors and friends, Jay Abraham, the nation's marketing guru, and Michael Levine, author, commentator and public relations consultant. The idea torrents keep flowing from these smart fellows.

Big thanks to Alan Gadney and Carolyn Porter of One-On-One Book Production and Marketing, who transformed this book from manuscript, through galley, to the finished product. And to Meryl Moss, public relations, for making the world aware of it.

Dan Poynter and John Kremer. Always generous with their time and sage advice. The small publisher's best friends.

Lindsey Kotler, Marketing Director of Ernest Mitchell Publishers. "Linds" put the myriad pieces together and faultlessly carried the ball from inception to completion. Makes her dad very proud.

# AUTHOR'S INTRODUCTION

Cosmetic surgery is now big. According to the American Society of Plastic Surgeons, in 2004, U.S. surgeons performed nearly 11.9 million surgical and non-surgical cosmetic procedures.

Cosmetic surgery's exposure has spread to a broader range of the public, creating a greater appreciation for the specialty's capabilities. There is plenty of talk about cosmetic surgery around the water cooler these days and much of it stems from the attention given to it by the media. "Reality Television" has embraced cosmetic surgery with *Extreme Makeover, The Swan, Nip/Tuck, Miami Slice* and, of course, my favorite, *Dr. 90210*. The subject has been brought into the homes of millions of people who had little prior knowledge but harbored a yearning to have their appearance improved. So the cat is out of the bag. But that also presents a challenge for those who are interested in cosmetic surgery because they need more information than they can glean from the snippets shown on television. They need solid, reliable information. Where does one go for information? How does one research the subject? And then there is the issue of "how far do you go" to see a cosmetic surgeon. Where you live may or may not have someone who has the credentials, experience and talent that you would prefer. There are advantages and disadvantages to traveling for cosmetic surgery. But in any event, whether you decide to have it close to home or in another location, you need a guide, a tutorial for getting a grip on how to select the right doctor and procedure for you. Because it is complex and because cosmetic surgery is not something you do every day, you do not have the necessary experience to make the best decision by yourself. There are dire consequences of poor decision making. Not only is there the issue of how well the procedure will turn out, but there are crucial safety issues as almost all procedures require anesthesia.

The quality of the result is proportional to the homework you do. If you select a doctor only from his or her listing in the phone directory, your prospects for satisfaction are not great. If you have an outline for investigating and interviewing, and apply that plan consistently and objectively, you will stand an excellent chance of selecting the most appropriate doctor. That is why you need a checklist, or better yet, checklists. When we surveyed readers of my last book, *SECRETS OF A BEVERLY HILLS COSMETIC SURGEON, The Expert's Guide to Safe, Successful Surgery*, the feature frequently cited as the most valuable was "the lists of questions."

Prospective cosmetic surgery patients quickly realize they are sailing through uncharted waters.

You have a lot to learn. But learn you must. You need to gather information so that you can make the best decision possible. Invoke the general rule of life: He or she who has the most accurate information makes the best decision. To help you, I have created this unique helper, a workbook of sorts. A book that makes you work. Interactive. A primer that raises your cosmetic surgery IQ by forcing you to perform an exercise. To recognize and digest questions that you need to pose at the consultation.

You must take this guidebook to your consultations or your time will be wasted. This workbook only works if you work with it. Open the book and then test the doctor. Not a test of cell biology or the biochemistry of antibiotics, but a test to determine compatibility. Does the doctor's education, training, experience and practice profile match your desires and needs? You do not need to be an MD or PhD to figure it out. Just follow this book's road map.

When used faithfully and consistently, this book will draw you, nearly on automatic pilot, to the right office. The technique of asking each prospective cosmetic surgeon the same question is borrowed from classic business-world hiring practices. Experienced job interviewers prepare a list of written questions to ask every interviewee. Only then can there be an objective, meaningful sorting and ranking of the candidates. That consistent process of asking the same questions makes any selection process more apt to be successful. The more data and the less emotion, the better.

> *An educated patient is a happy patient. The more you, the patient, understand about cosmetic surgery, the better decision you will make when determining what is the right choice and the right procedure for you.*
>
> **— Angela O'Mara, President The Professional Image, Inc. Cosmetic Surgery Magazine, October 1999**

Finally, many of the questions I suggest you ask were originally posed to me by patients. As patients learn from doctors, doctors learn from patients. I want you to learn a lot from this doctor. After all, the word *doctor*, from the Latin word *docere*, means to teach.

## Being a Well-Informed Patient Is a Plus for the Patient and the Doctor

I've been asked by a few patients whether bringing this guide to the consultation would somehow be considered by the doctor to be inappropriate. Would he feel he's in competition with "a cosmetic surgeon he's never met and who's written a book?" And would he think he's being unfairly put on the spot?

In my experience, the best, most enlightened physicians appreciate a well-informed, well-prepared patient. They do not feel threatened. They welcome the opportunity to answer well-thought-out questions with forthright answers. Furthermore, when the patient comes to the consultation with a focused and structured agenda, the doctor's time is used well, not wasted. It's frustrating to be ready to answer any and all questions, only to be faced with a patient who is scattered and can't seem to zero in on the issues at hand. When the patient and the doctor are respectful of each other's time and intelligence, everyone benefits.

> *Interest in cosmetic plastic surgery is at an all-time high. Because of this high level of interest, and the amount of sometimes confusing information, the need to have better informed cosmetic plastic surgery patients has never been greater.*
> **— James H. Wells, MD, FACS
> President of the American
> Society of Plastic Surgeons
> 2002-2003**

## Make This Book Work for You

You are the best arbiter of what is comfortable and appropriate for you. If you'd rather not have this book in hand at your consultation, feel free to write the relevant questions in your own hand in a notebook. Or photocopy the pages that deal with your procedure and bring those with you. I want this book to work for you, so I'm happy to give you free access to any part of it and encourage you to use it to your best advantage.

## Every Word in This Book Was Written by Me

Because I like to write conversationally (I was once dubbed "The King of Run-On Sentences"), my unedited written sentences tend to be long. Too long for the tough editors who shape up the text. But they only edit; I write. What you read here are my thoughts, my words. Not those of a writer-for-hire or a co-author (who does 95 percent of the writing) or a ghost writer. You are hearing from me — a practicing cosmetic surgeon for more than 35 years — who consults and operates five days a week. Today, no time for golf; maybe someday. But not now. I still have serious work to do and I have a passion for teaching — teaching you.

---

Dr. Michael Schwartz, a Pasadena, California, surgeon: "Surgical advances, improved technology and developments in anesthesiology, which make cosmetic surgery safer and more affordable to the general public, also make it more socially acceptable. Patients no longer have to go into postoperative hibernation for a month. Now they return to work and resume their lives almost immediately, in some cases as if nothing has happened, in other cases, eager to proselytize about what has happened."

**— Ellen Feldman**
**"Before and After"**
*American Heritage*, **February/March 2004**

---

# PROGRAM NOTES

Before we start, a couple of program notes. I cannot cover all details and technicalities of all the procedures within the realm of cosmetic surgery. My scope is limited to the fourteen most common, effective, well-established core procedures. The important ones that make big differences. **Appendix C** lists them in a spreadsheet format for an at-a-glance review.

Patient comments, interspersed throughout the text, are quoted verbatim from written notes and letters received by us. To protect patient confidentiality, complete identification is not provided.

Finally, in referring to doctors, patients and others, I shall use "he." This is not to imply that there are not female doctors; of course there are. Because it is somewhat cumbersome to constantly use "he or she," as a matter of routine, the masculine gender will be employed. No sexism. Just word economy.

> *You don't have to be young to be youthful.*
> **— Bernice Rosen**
> **Los Angeles**
> **Age indeterminate**

Any good plastic surgeon *is* and **must be** a psychologist, whether he would have it so or not. when you change a man's face, you almost invariably change his future. Change his physical image, and nearly always you change the man — his personality, his behavior — and sometimes even his basic talents and abilities.

**— Maxwell Maltz, MD, FICS**
*Psycho-Cybernetics, A New*
*Way to Get More Living out of Life*

# 1

# COSMETIC SURGERY —
# *What It Can and Cannot Do*

## Are You REALLY a Candidate?
## These 15 Scenarios and Comments Will Tell You

Cosmetic surgery is not for just anyone. Since this is a book of questions, here are 15 sample reasons you might have for cosmetic surgery. The comments will help answer your question: *are you or are you not an appropriate candidate?*

1.  **You wish to improve your appearance because:**
    your mirror is demonstrating signs of aging:
    baggy eyes, jowls, double chin, wrinkled face, sagging breasts, jodhpur hips.

2.  **Certain physical features are unsatisfying to you:**
    prominent nose, receding chin, low eyebrows, small breasts, disproportionately large breasts, over-plump buttocks, flanks or hips, or flank fat rolls that defy diet and exercise, wrinkled skin, jowls, sagging neck, double chin.

3.  **You are a mother of three, and your breasts and tummy sag despite a vigorous workout schedule.**

4. Your lips are thin.

5. Your upper eyelids droop, but you are not necessarily tired.

   **Comment:** Numbers 1, 2, 3, 4 and 5 represent valid indications for cosmetic surgery.

6. You are unhappy with your social life and believe a new look can invigorate it.

7. You are recently divorced and anxious to "hook up" with someone and are convinced a new look will enhance your prospects.

8. You are overweight and hope liposuction will give you a "quick fix."

   **Comment:** Numbers 6, 7 and 8 deal with issues for which cosmetic surgery is not a satisfactory answer.

9. **You are in the entertainment world.** You are not getting the roles you want and think cosmetic surgery will help.

10. **You are a model** and your agent suggests that "you are great, but your nose is too big."

11. **Your career is stagnant.** Your occupation is populated by younger people and you sense there is a career advantage to looking younger and not shopworn.

    **Comment:** Numbers 9, 10 and 11 require some additional thought and explanation. Number 9 deals with people seeking certain roles in the entertainment world. What you have to ask yourself, your agent and the people with whom you interact, is whether or not it is realistic to expect that more parts will be available to you if certain features are changed. The same logic applies to Number 10. Often, casting directors and modeling agency directors cannot be certain that a change in a physical feature will assure further work assignments.

---

Q: If a Hollywood actress is revealed to have had plastic surgery, will it hurt her career?

A: No, says one top Hollywood casting director. "It's about what you look like. Plastic surgery doesn't compromise your career as long as you look good and sexy. We don't care how you got there, as long as you got there."

— **"The Big Question"**
*Star*, **January 3, 2005**

---

**Comment:** Number 11 is the most intriguing. It is a fact that an employer may choose the more youthful and energetic-looking candidate for a specific position. Certainly, experience is to be valued, but unfortunately experience alone may not be enough. The combination of a youthful appearance plus experience is ideal.

---

In the Seventh Annual Kennedy-Krannich Career Book Picks of the Year, Joyce Kennedy of Tribune Media Services, chose as one of its 10 selections for 2003, *SECRETS OF A BEVERLY HILLS COSMETIC SURGEON, The Expert's Guide to Safe, Successful Surgery.* In informing us of this honor, Joyce wrote:

> *It is not really a stretch to be included in the list of the 10 best career books of the year because age is taking a big hit in the job market. The book is terrific and will help more people than you may ever know.*

In Joyce's column announcing the winners, she described the book as: the ultimate guide to erecting a (job) bias defense shield. The author knows every wrinkle (pardon) ever erased to keep you looking young and vibrant in the job market.

---

12. **Your five-year-old tells you your nose is too big.**

13. **You are a 15-year-old young lady** and your grandmother keeps asking you: "When are you going to go see a cosmetic surgeon about your nose?"

    **Comment:** Numbers 12 and 13 deal with the opinions others have of your physical features. Their opinions are not important; what is important is your opinion. Make the decision for yourself, for reasons that are important to you and not to satisfy someone else.

14. **You are 69 years old.** You have had three facelifts, two eyelid surgeries and a chemical skin peel. Your friends and family tell you "you look terrific." A movie theater cashier demands Medicare card or proof of age when you request a senior discount. But at cocktail parties, you accost a cosmetic surgeon and obsess about "these lines around my eyes."

    **Comment:** Number 14 deals with a common scenario: people become obsessed and focus on the barely visible and/or unimportant. What counts is the total appearance. A line or two here does not make for an aged face. No go.

15. **You are a high-profile media personality and your face is recognized by millions of people.** You have had so much cosmetic facial surgery you are developing a strange, monkey-like look. Yet, you "want more."

**Comment:** Number 15 is a reminder that there is a pool of quicksand that awaits those who seek to go beyond a reasonable cosmetic surgery expectation. I don't have to remind you of the celebrities who unfortunately fell into that quicksand and never got their faces out.

The above are common and classic consultation comments. All have been excerpted from actual consultations. Which of these 15 scenarios match your motivations and desires? Which are healthy? Which are unwise and potentially risky?

> *The young want to be older and the older want to be younger. It's just another chapter in Americans' endless happiness.*
> **— Robert J. Samuelson**
> **"Ventures in Agelessness"**
> *Newsweek*, **November 3, 2003**

# 2

# THE SEVEN KEY QUESTIONS YOU MUST ASK YOURSELF

**B**elow are the seven issues and concerns most frequently shared with us by prospective patients. It may be that one or more are also your concerns. *Everyone* has concerns.

| CONCERN | LEVEL OF CONCERN | |
|---|---|---|
| | Major | Minor |
| **1.** I'm afraid. The idea of any surgery and/or anesthesia scares me. | ☐ | ☐ |
| **2.** What will I look like? Will I be happy with the result? Will it look natural? | ☐ | ☐ |
| **3.** How long before I can return to social activities, work or exercise? | ☐ | ☐ |
| **4.** Will it be painful? | ☐ | ☐ |
| **5.** What will my family, friends or even coworkers think about this? | ☐ | ☐ |
| **6.** Can I afford what I want? | ☐ | ☐ |
| **7.** Which doctor is best qualified for my particular case? | ☐ | ☐ |

*Cosmetic surgery has become very popular, especially with the baby boomers. It has become more accepted and certainly easier to obtain. With all of this expansion come more potential problems. Mass advertising and lack of enforceable regulations have led to irresponsible behavior on the part of some physicians. If you are considering having anything done you need to research and become an informed patient.*

**— Susan Fontana**
**"Whose Hands Do I Choose? Part 2"**
*Cosmetic Surgery News*, **October 2003**

# 3

# THE MOST IMPORTANT DECISION — *DOCTOR SELECTION*

### A Little Secret:
### Just Because It Says "Plastic Surgery" or "Cosmetic Surgery" on the Door
### Doesn't Mean You're in the Right Place

Cosmetic surgery is always elective (not essential to life) surgery. You have the luxury of time to make the best decision possible. The challenge you will face is finding, managing and interpreting all the information available.

One reliable route for choosing a cosmetic surgeon is through a recommendation from a friend or acquaintance pleased with his or her surgery's result. If a person is willing to share that they have had cosmetic surgery, he or she will usually be equally willing to discuss the entire experience. Be careful to compare the procedure you are considering with the one they have had. Remember, compare "nose to nose," "breasts to breasts." Don't assume a successful breast surgery guarantees the expertise demanded for a nose job. Different territory, different techniques.

The ideal medical referral sources are surgeons, operating room nurses, surgical technicians and anesthesia specialists. Those who actually see the cosmetic surgeon performing his craft in the operating room are the most useful witnesses. Those are the "experts" I contact if I'm checking out a surgeon for family or a friend.

## My Four Key Criteria in Identifying a Top Cosmetic Surgeon:

- ☞ **Board certification**\* in one of the four specialties that legitimately and routinely perform cosmetic procedures within their defined scope of practice: dermatology, head and neck surgery, ophthalmology and plastic surgery.

- ☞ **Fellowship training** in the cosmetic surgery of the doctor's board-certified specialty.

- ☞ **Medical school teaching appointment.**

- ☞ **Practices cosmetic surgery exclusively** – no reconstruction, e.g., burns or hand surgery, accidents, cancer surgery, birth defects. One hundred percent focus on cosmetic surgery!

I just made the sorting a lot simpler for you.

## NOTE: A Quick Way to Compare Cosmetic Surgeons on Paper

When comparing surgeons, place their respective professional biographies side by side. The focused cosmetic surgeon's professional history will be replete with references to cosmetic surgery training, experience, research and teaching. A surgeon who does not specialize exclusively in cosmetic surgery may be stronger in other work: cancer, reconstruction, trauma or birth defects. Add this information to what you

---

\*   See Chapter 10, **"Homework,"** for more information on the specialty boards and how to contact them to confirm board certification.

gather through friends, medical personnel and your office visit and you will be well on your way to short-listing the best surgeon for your needs.

*Once you have done your research and selected a physician for a consultation, you need to be prepared with a list of questions. The written list is extremely important because it is very easy to feel intimidated and forget what you want to ask.*

— **Susan Fontana**
**"Whose Hands Do I Choose? Part 2"**
**Cosmetic Surgery News, October 2003**

## Characteristics of a Physician — Good and Bad

| Ideal Characteristics | Undesirable Characteristics |
| --- | --- |
| Communicative | Hurried |
| Caring | Doesn't care |
| Takes time | Arrogant |
| Competent | Inattentive |
| Listens | Kept me waiting |
| Friendly | Doesn't explain enough |
| Thoroughly interested | Careless with prescriptions |
| Sincere | Ineffective treatment |
| Prompt | Reluctant to refer or consult |

Source: *Journal of Health Care Marketing*, June 1986

# 4

# ALWAYS SEEK A COSMETIC SURGERY *SUPERSPECIALIST*

## *You Don't Have to Go to Beverly Hills*

### Why Superspecialization?

The history of surgery is one of continual progress made through increasingly narrow specialization by its practitioners. Only 88 years ago, there were no specialties within surgery itself. All surgery – from brain to toe – was done by "a surgeon." And then, that "surgeon" had no formal specialty training after medical school. But today's medical education trend is to train doctors who will be more skillful in a relatively limited portion of the body. A "jack of all trades, master of none" is not satisfactory in today's highly specialized medical world. There are great benefits to patients when a surgeon narrows his scope and chooses not to perform most other operations within his specialty. Now there are eye surgeons who limit their practice to the retina, chest surgeons who perform only open-heart procedures, and orthopedic surgeons who do only knee surgery.

This fine honing of specialization in modern medical practice is known as *superspecialization*: a narrow, focused, "boutique" practice. Great benefits to the patient are realized when a surgeon narrows his scope and concentrates on a limited selection of procedures.

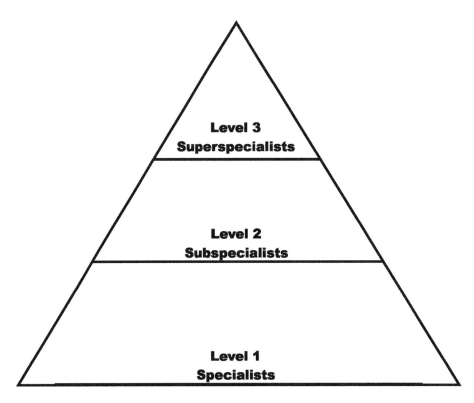

**Cosmetic Surgery Hierarchy**
*The Hierarchy of Modern Medical Superspecialization*

**Level 1:** *Specialist.* Some cosmetic surgery but most time spent on reconstructive surgery for disease or accident. Board certified. No fellowship training.

**Level 2:** *Subspecialist.* Practices both reconstructive and cosmetic procedures, but not the full scope of the parent specialty. Typically board certified plus fellowship training beyond his residency.

**Level 3:** *Superspecialist.* Practices cosmetic surgery exclusively. No reconstructive surgery. Typically board certified and fellowship trained, the most specialized of all practitioners. In the world of cosmetic surgery, these doctors are at the apex of sophistication, training and skill.

Superspecialists are the product of post-residency fellowship training, and the importance of such fellowships cannot be underestimated. The refinement and focus of subspecialty education will continue to narrow as we recognize that achieving surgical excellence requires a depth of knowledge that is more valuable than mere width.

By now you should have no doubt that the more specialized the doctor, the greater the likelihood of good results for you, the patient. You now know that if you are considering a facelift, you should seek a board certified specialist who performs only cosmetic surgery and has served a cosmetic surgery fellowship. A cosmetic surgery superspecialist will typically limit his practice to 15 or fewer procedures mastered after lifelong study, focus and dedication.

Patients do understand, instinctively, the importance of choosing a doctor whose focus matches their specific need. We now hear patients say with increasing frequency: "I want a cosmetic surgeon who doesn't do *everything*." The public has endorsed superspecialization by increasingly patronizing the more specialized and focused doctors. It makes sense, doesn't it?

*According to James Carraway, MD, a plastic surgeon in Virginia Beach, Virginia, training is critical, in cosmetic surgeons – regardless of their titles – must spend years honing their craft in order to keep patients happy with outcomes. "Every patient wants a home run," Dr. Carraway stated. "Not a double or triple. Training is what differentiates cosmetic surgeons," he says.*
— **Cosmetic Surgery Times, August 2004**

# 5

# THE SCREENING CALL

## *A Five-Minute Call Can Save You Two Hours and $200*

This is one of my favorite tactics to save you time and money. Why take precious hours and hard-earned dollars to visit a doctor who turns out to be inappropriate — for whatever reason — for your needs?

Instead, once you have a list of prospective cosmetic surgeons, make a few two-minute calls. You could save hours and hundreds of dollars.

A few tips to remember before you call:

- Ask for the office manager; go straight to the top. He will always be the most knowledgeable.

- Call at 9 a.m. The manager is fresh and will have more time to chat.

- Stick to my script. Don't go off on tangents. Don't start asking technical questions about your sister-in-law's breast surgery experience. Remember, you have only one aim:  to decide if a particular practice is worthy of a consultation. Get on with the task at hand.

*Finding the right doctor is more confusing now than it ever was.*

> — **Mark L. Jewell, MD**
> **President of the American Society for**
> **Aesthetic Plastic Surgery,** *NewBeauty Magazine* January 2005

The following checklist will be your outline for a productive, efficient phone inquiry.

## Checklist for Telephone Screening Call:

Name of doctor: _____

Address: _____

Phone: _____

Questions to ask:

✔ Is the doctor board certified?  If the answer is "yes," which specialty board? The American Board of _____.

See Chapter 10, **"Homework"** for more information on the four recognized boards whose diplomates have met the standards of the profession as  fully qualified specialists.

✔ Did the doctor serve a cosmetic surgery fellowship?

✔ Does the practice conduct cosmetic surgery only?

Time out. If, so far, you don't have at least two "yes" answers, say: "Thank you, good-bye" and go on to the next doctor on the list. That practice was not for you.

✔ What five procedures does the doctor perform most frequently?  If what you're considering doesn't make the list, say "Good-bye."

✔ Where does the doctor perform his surgeries?  Office? Outpatient surgery center?  Hospital? (circle response).

✔ Is office or outpatient surgery center facility **licensed by the state, certified by Medicare** and/or accredited by **JCAHO, AAAASF or AAAHC?**∗ *(circle one or more). If none of the above, you are courting danger. Tell the  manager your sink is overflowing and hang up.*

∗ See Chapter 10, "**Homework**" for more information on surgical facility accrediting organizations.

✔ Anesthesia.

If administered by a board-certified anesthesiologist, who further specializes in cosmetic surgery, give the practice an "A" in Anesthesia.

If by a nurse-anesthetist, ask if he is supervised by a board-certified anesthesiologist. If so, grade the practice "A-." If no supervision, "B."

If the surgeon is administering the anesthetic, that's like asking a jockey to ride two horses simultaneously. Give the practice an "F" for Fail and hang up quickly!

✔ What is the cost for the procedure(s) being considered?

Ask if all services are included: surgery center, anesthesia specialist, recovery hideaway (if appropriate), medications. You need to know if your budget is in the ballpark. While an exact charge may depend on particulars of your case, a fee range or most common fee should be given by the manager.

If the practice won't reveal any significant fee information over the phone, why waste time consulting with a doctor who may not be affordable?  It's like ogling the cars at the Mercedes dealership when your budget says Ford Taurus.

✔ What is the consultation fee?  $_____.
Is that charge applicable to the surgical fee?

✔ Will the consultation include computer imaging?  While many excellent cosmetic surgeons do not use this stunning tool, I believe a consultation without it has less value (see Chapter 6 **"Treat the Consultation as a Job Interview"** for more information on computer imaging).

*Going on a consultation for cosmetic surgery can be intimidating. It is important to be prepared and have completed most of your research before you go. There is no point in going on numerous consultations only to later find out the credentials of the surgeons aren't acceptable. The importance of evaluating a physician's credentials cannot be overemphasized.*

— **Susan Fontana**
**"Whose Hands Do I Choose? Part 2"**
*Cosmetic Surgery News***, October 2003**

# What Else Reveals That You're Speaking to a Great Office?

When I call a professional office, within the first 20 seconds I can sense whether or not I am speaking with a high-quality, service-oriented, sharp practice. Here are my criteria for excellence:

☎ The call is answered after no more than four rings.

☎ You should never get a busy signal.

☎ You are greeted by a warm, courteous, cheery, glad-to-be-of-service staff member. You can almost see the smile through the telephone line.

☎ The person answering your call is knowledgeable, helpful and able to answer most or all questions promptly. You sense that she has been well trained to help and educate you.
What you don't want to hear is, "Gee, I don't know," and then a long pause.

☎ If there is a question she cannot answer, you are promptly transferred to another staff member who is qualified and who can answer it.

☎ You are offered additional, complementary teaching aids, e.g., brochures, pamphlets, video- or audiotapes, etc. These further explain the services available to you. And, they will be U.S. mailed, e-mailed, or faxed promptly. Most surgeons provide prospective patients with appropriate brochures and pamphlets prior to the consultation. This allows the patient to review important points about the procedure(s) under consideration. Being prepared in advance guarantees a more productive session with the doctor. Questions raised while reading this material can be answered during the consultation.

☎ If you decide to schedule a consultation, you are offered several choices for your convenience.

☎ The date and time are confirmed with you prior to the conversation's end. You also are assured that you will receive a written confirmation, including directions to the office and parking advice.

☎ As the conversation ends, you are reminded of the name or names of the staff members with whom you spoke. You are encouraged to call them if you have any further questions. These are your "contact" people.

☎ If you ask about fees, you receive some meaningful information. While an exact fee quotation requires a consultation and evaluation by the doctor, a superior office will offer a "range of fees" or "most common fee" for the procedure or procedures you are interested in. You have the right to know so you can evaluate whether your budget is "in the ballpark."

☎ Finally, the office will ask for your daytime and evening phone numbers so you can be contacted several days prior to your consultation. They will want to be certain you received the promised information and also confirm the appointment particulars. Having your phone numbers also allows the office to inform you should any change in the office's schedule affect your appointment time.

Is all this important? I think so. Consider yourself a customer; you want good service.

Service begins with that first telephone call. Every practice takes its cues from the top; the doctor sets the standards; it is his practice; he is the boss.

The doctor must care about you, the caller, before he ever meets you. If not, if he does not have in place smart, able and conscientious staff "up front," how particular, how attentive and how competent might he and his team be in the operating room and during the recovery phase? Think about it. Always opt for quality; you don't have cosmetic surgery every day.

---

*You need to take your time, come up with a plan and be disciplined in following it.*

**— Susan Fontana**
**"Whose Hands Do I Choose? Part 2"**
***Cosmetic Surgery News*, October 2003**

# 6

# TREAT THE CONSULTATION AS A JOB INTERVIEW
## *You're Hiring a Surgeon*

### Before the Consultation

- When you schedule your consultation, be as specific as you can about your desires. For example, if you are consulting because you had an unsuccessful nasal surgery previously, please tell the staff member. Why? Because that will trigger some responses from them that can optimize the value of your consultation, and make it more efficient. Hearing that you wish to discuss a possible second surgery, you will be advised to bring copies of your medical records and photographs from your first surgery (you can get them easily by calling or writing to your previous surgeon's office). Having all your records will help the consulting doctor give his best recommendation at your first meeting.

- You will get more out of the consultation by preparing for it. Study the educational materials the doctor has sent you in response to your initial call for information. Write down the questions you wish to ask.

**Your surgeon should:**

Answer all of your questions thoroughly and clearly

Ask for your reaction to recommendations

Offer alternatives, where appropriate, without pressuring you to consider unneeded or additional procedures

Welcome questions about professional qualifications, experience, costs and payment policies

Make clear the risks of surgery and possible outcomes

Give you information about the surgery you want

Leave the final decision to you

You also have the right to expect that your surgery will take place in a surgical facility or hospital that is safe and well equipped. Facilities with accreditation from a recognized accrediting organization have demonstrated that they have appropriate equipment and staff to safely monitor patients and deal with potential complications.

**— American Society for Aesthetic Plastic Surgery**

## Practical Consultation Hints

● **Bring a friend or relative with you.** "Four ears and four eyes are twice as good for learning." Your companion may see or hear something that you may miss. The idea is to leave the consultation armed with as much information as possible.

● **Take notes.** Write down the responses/answers to this book's questions. Then you can leisurely review them at home. *Compare the answers to the same questions posed to different doctors.* This book is your personal cosmetic surgery consultation journal. Use it well. Don't save it for the bookshelf. Write in it!

*Communication is the key. Visual aides, particularly a photo gallery of typical results from cosmetic surgery, can help demonstrate what is possible or not possible. Viewing photographs of "real" people who have undergone plastic surgery can help bring patients back down to earth.*

**— Stanley A. Klatsky, MD**
**Editorial, "What Patients Want"**
***Aesthetic Surgery Journal*, September/October 2003**

● **Request a take-home copy of the computer imaging "before and after."** Either on disc or as a hard copy. Review at your leisure.

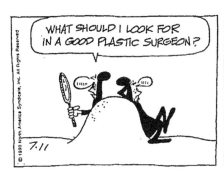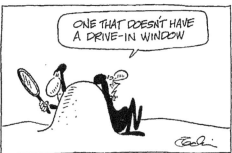

## If a Cosmetic Surgeon Proposes a "New" Procedure or Product
### Better Ask Some Questions

Science never sleeps. Every day medical science progresses, even cosmetic surgery. Many procedures, techniques, drugs and products I routinely use today were unknown even 10 years ago. That's the good news.

The bad news is that in today's fast-paced world, with hordes of hungry-for-a-story media folks, the "latest" or "newest" operation or product, lip filler or wrinkle eraser is given immediate exposure and attention and, hence, some credibility and even popularity. Often, in my opinion, way too soon. Often, they come to market unproven.

In the world of cosmetic procedures, it takes years before all the benefits — and all the complications and dissatisfactions — come to awareness. We don't have the privilege of working out the details by testing on baboons in the animal lab. Many of the first patients to have these procedures performed on them or new materials injected into them, will experience some unhappiness, dissatisfaction or worse.

That is why, for the benefit of my patients, I am never the "first kid on the block" to implement "the latest." Maybe it's my inbred Midwestern conservatism, but I prefer the test of time. I'll let other doctors and their often unwitting patients "show me the way," thereby demonstrating what *really* happens in the long run. Because, it is the long run that counts in cosmetic surgery. Most of what we do is intended to be semi-permanent, to last many, many years. That creates a burden that says what we do not only has to be good but safe, predictable and, hopefully, long lasting.

In the mythical race between cosmetic surgery tortoises and hares, I prefer to bet on the slow but steady. As doctors, it's no fun to preside over a complication or to listen to the complaints and unhappiness of a dissatisfied patient. Our mission is to make people happy.

To summarize, my advice: ***Caveat Emptor!*** Buyer beware.

> *As major new medical technology is developed and made available for use, its worth is measured on the basis of the value and safety it confers on patients. Part of the process of evaluation should include a comparison with existing and proven technologies that deal with similar clinical problems. The qualifications of those who propose to use the new technologies must be carefully assessed, verifying that the individual has had comprehensive education...and has acquired the necessary technical skills and is competent to recognize and manage any complications resulting from use of the new technology.*
>
> **— Committee on Emerging Surgical Technology and Education
> of the American College of Surgeons, June 1995**

> *Too often, marketing can drown out medical science.*
>
> **— James F. Fries, MD
> Stanford University
> — quoted in *The New York Times*, December 19, 2004**

Here is my short list of questions you want to ask if you are considering having the procedure you just saw premiered on the local news, *Prime Time* or *60 Minutes*, or after your doctor says: "Try this, it's brand new."

Those short snappy questions may not be what the doctor is used to hearing. But they empower you — not the doctor's ego or pride — and that is what's important.

When you weigh and analyze the answers, you'll make a better decision. ***I guarantee it.***

# Checklist for New Procedure(s):

✔ How long has the procedure been performed in the U.S.?

✔ Doctor, how long have you been performing it?

✔ How many times have you performed the procedure?

✔ What is the longest case follow- up you have had?

✔ May I see before-and-after photos of typical results?

✔ May I speak with a patient who had this performed recently?

✔ May I know the name of the surgeon who originated the technique?

✔ Which other cosmetic surgeons in this community perform the same procedure?

✔ What are the possible complications, side effects, dissatisfactions?

✔ Of these, which is the most common complication?

✔ Which is the most serious?

✔ If complications occur or I'm dissatisfied, how can this be corrected? And are there additional costs for the correction?

## Business Issues

Before you sign up for cosmetic surgery, you need to be comfortable with all the costs. No guesswork, no surprises, no "add-ons." As you consult and collect fee quotes, be sure you know *exactly* what services are — and are not — included, and how you pay for these services.

Here's my list of "must ask" questions. Don't be embarrassed to ask any of these. It's your money; you work hard for it.

# Business Issues Checklist

**Always ask: "What is the *total cost*." Does this include:**

- ✔ Surgery facility charges?
- ✔ Anesthesia specialist's fee?
- ✔ Recovery hideaway (if appropriate) charge?
- ✔ Medications, dressing supplies?
- ✔ Touch-up procedures?
- ✔ Assuming a scheduling fee or deposit is required to reserve a surgery date, is it fully or partially refundable if I change my mind? How much notice need I give?

**Do you accept credit cards?**

**Are insurance benefits available?**  Note: Nasal surgery for breathing problems, breast reduction to relieve pain and back problems, and upper eyelid surgery, to correct obscured vision, are the most likely to qualify.

**If the procedure is insurance-eligible:**

- ✔ Do you bill the insurance company on my behalf?
- ✔ Do you "accept assignment," i.e., payment made directly to doctor?
- ✔ Is a deposit required?
- ✔ What if insurance pays nothing?  Or poorly?  Will you help with my appeal?  If so, exactly what will you or your office do?

**Compare financing plans:**

- ✔ Application form online?
- ✔ In office?
- ✔ Maximum amount financed?
- ✔ Interest rate, APR?
- ✔ Grace period?
- ✔ Payment to patient or MD?
- ✔ Is there a charge-back to the doctor's office? That could increase your cost.

(See **Appendix C** – "Companies that Finance Cosmetic Surgery")

Questions to ask concerning a possible discount or courtesy fee reduction:

✔ Do you offer a "standby" fee?

✔ Are there "friends and family" group discounts?

✔ Do you have a "layaway" plan discount?

Americans spent just under $9.4 billion on cosmetic procedures; this figure does not include fees for surgical facilities, anesthesia, medical tests, prescriptions, surgical garments or other miscellaneous expenses associated with surgery. Six and a half billion dollars were for surgical procedures, and $2.9 billion for nonsurgical procedures.

**— News Release**
*American Society for Aesthetic Plastic Surgery (ASAPS), 2004 Statistics,*
*February 2005*

# CHECKLISTS FOR THE 14 MOST COMMON PROCEDURES:

## *The Crucial Questions to Ask*

### BODY PROCEDURES

Breast Augmentation

Breast Lift

Breast Reduction

Liposuction

Tummy Tuck

### FACE & NECK PROCEDURES

Cheek Implants

Chin Augmentation

Correction of Protruding Ears

Eyelid Surgery

Face & Neck Lift

Facial Rejuvenation: Laser or Chemical

Forehead & Eyebrow Lift

Nasal Surgery

Neck Sculpture

---

The top five surgical procedures for women were: liposuction, breast augmentation, eyelid surgery, tummy tuck and facelift.

The top five surgical procedures for men were: liposuction, eyelid surgery, rhinoplasty, male breast reduction and hair transplantation.

**American Society for Aesthetic Plastic Surgery, 2004 Statistics, February 2005**

---

# BODY PROCEDURES

**AUTHOR'S NOTE:** *Because I perform cosmetic surgery on the face and neck only, I am not an expert on body sculpture procedures: breast surgery, liposuction, or tummy tucks. The basic information I present to you, in this chapter, was gleaned from the excellent public education brochures provided by the American Society of Plastic Surgeons.*

## BREAST AUGMENTATION*
### *(Augmentation Mammaplasty)*

Your plastic surgeon performs breast augmentation using implants made of medical grade, biocompatible, textured or smooth silicone shells filled with sterile saline solution. Should the implant rupture or leak, the saline is safely absorbed by the body and poses no health hazard. Implants may be prefilled prior to placement, or slowly filled at the time of the surgery through a self-sealing valve. Implant placement, type and size is determined based on your breast anatomy, body type and desired increase in size, as well as your plastic surgeon's judgment. Implant manufacturers occasionally introduce new styles and types of implants; there may be additional options available to you, including silicone-gel-filled implants.

Breast implants have not been shown to impair breast health. Careful review of scientific research by independent groups such as the National Academy of Sciences Institute of Medicine (IOM) has found no proven link between breast implants and autoimmune or other systemic diseases in women. Implants can, however, create subtle or more noticeable changes in the look and feel of your breasts. Capsular contracture, a condition that causes the naturally forming scar tissue around a breast implant to contract, occurs in a variable percentage of patients and can make the breast feel firmer than normal. While this condition can be addressed surgically, correction is not always permanent.

---

\* Les Bolton, MD, FACS, of the Cosmetic Surgery Specialists Group of Beverly Hills, Clinical Instructor of Plastic Surgery, USC School of Medicine and Diplomate of the American Board of Plastic Surgery, contributed to this section.

Questions about any breast procedure or breast implants and related topics of health can be found at the Medical library resource of the U.S. National Institutes of Health, http://www.nlm.nih.gov/medlineplus/breastimplants breastreconstruction.html

You should be aware that breast implants are not guaranteed to last a lifetime, and that future surgery may be required to replace one or both implants. Pregnancy, weight loss and menopause may influence the appearance of augmented breasts over the course of a woman's lifetime. Breast augmentation requires maintenance over time, including regular examinations for breast health and to evaluate the condition of your implants.

A mammogram or CT scan may be recommended prior to your procedure to ensure breast health and serve as a baseline for future comparison. Following the procedure, X-ray studies are technically more difficult. Obtaining the best possible results requires specialized techniques and additional views. You must be candid about your implants when undergoing any diagnostic breast exam.

Breast procedures should be performed only by a surgeon certified by the American Board of Plastic Surgery. No other medical specialty includes formal training and testing to maintain credentials in all breast procedures.
— *NewBeauty Magazine*
**January 2005**

# BREAST AUGMENTATION

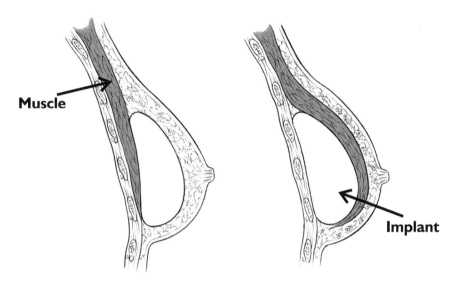

Muscle

Implant

**Placement superficial to muscle**     **Placement deep to muscle**

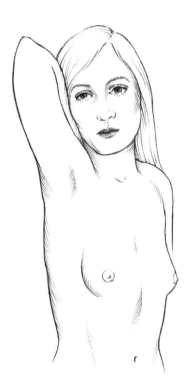

**Doctor: indicate incision location**

# Breast Augmentation Checklist

✔ Silicone-filled implants look and feel very natural. They were once thought to be associated with unusual autoimmune diseases until scientific studies proved otherwise. Can I have them if I want them?

_____

_____

✔ What type of implant do you recommend for me?

_____

_____

✔ What are the risks and complications associated with having breast implants?

_____

_____

✔ If my breasts are not symmetrical after surgery, what can be done?

_____

_____

✔ I have seen some implants that look very unnatural — they look like they are right under the skin. Is this condition a function of the type of implant, or its placement?

_____

_____

✔ If I do not want any visible scars, what is my best option?

_____

_____

✔ Is it dangerous to put implants under the chest muscle near the rib cage?

_____

_____

✔ I heal poorly, with thick scars. Is there a greater risk of capsule thickening for me?

_____

_____

✔ What shape, size, surface texturing, incision site and placement site is recommended for me?

_____

_____

✔ As I get older, will my breasts sag more with implants? If so, what can be done?

_____

_____

✔ If I gain weight and my breasts enlarge, will they become saggy?

_____

_____

✔ Will implants make it harder for my doctor to detect breast cancer?

_____

_____

✔ Do implants compromise the value of mammograms?

_____

_____

✔ What happens if an implant ruptures or leaks? How will I know? How will my breasts look? What can be done?

_____

_____

✔ If I get an infection, does the breast implant have to come out? What about the other implant? If it stays, will I look unnatural?

_____

_____

✔ After surgery, how long before I can engage in strenuous exercise?

_____

_____

✔ How long before I can have sex?

_____

_____

✔ What if I am not happy with the size of my implants?

_____

_____

✔ Can they be "exchanged"?

_____

_____

✔ What is the most common complication of breast enlargement?
How is this handled?

_____

_____

✔ What is the most serious complication?

_____

_____

✔ Some Hollywood people have obvious breast implants and look
grotesque. Do they look this way because of their own poor
judgment, the surgeon's judgment or a combination of both?

_____

_____

✔ Where will the incision be made?

_____

_____

✔ How can I expect my implanted breasts to look over time?

_____

_____

✔ Please tell me about the new breast implant via the belly button
operation.

_____

_____

✔ Can you give me information about the implant that I hear is
adjustable in size after surgery?

_____

_____

✔ What type of anesthesia is used? How long does the operation
take?

_____

_____

✔ How painful is this procedure?  How will the pain be controlled?
_____
_____

✔ How long will I be off work?
_____
_____

✔ If I have implants and become pregnant later, will the implants affect my baby and/or breast milk?
_____
_____

✔ How will my ability to breast-feed be affected?
_____
_____

✔ How can I expect my implanted breasts to look after pregnancy? After breast-feeding?
_____
_____

✔ Will I lose feeling of the breast or the nipple?
_____
_____

✔ Will breast implants correct sagging breasts?
_____
_____

✔ Will I have cleavage after the implants?
_____
_____

✔ Will my breasts become hard?
_____
_____

✔ How many additional operations on my implanted breast(s) can I expect during my lifetime?
_____
_____

✔ How will my breasts look if I decide to have the implants removed without replacement?

_____

_____

✔ What are my options if I am dissatisfied with the cosmetic outcome of my implanted breasts?

_____

_____

✔ Do I have to wear special bras?

_____

_____

✔ Do you have before-and-after photos I can look at for each procedure, and which results are reasonable for me?

_____

_____

✔ What alternate procedures or products are available if I choose not to have breast implants?

_____

_____

✔ On average, how many of these procedures do you perform annually?

_____

_____

✔ For this procedure, what percentage of your patients require a "touch-up" or "redo"?

_____

_____

# Notes:

_____

In 1961 Dr. Thomas Cronin unveiled a silicone implant, and the plastic surgery establishment and women across the land took it to their breasts.

**— Ellen Feldman**
**"Before and After"**
_American Heritage_, **February/March 2004**

# BREAST LIFT*
## (Mastopexy)

Breast lift is a highly individualized procedure achieved through a variety of incision patterns and techniques. The appropriate technique for your case will be determined based on:

- Breast size and shape
- The size and position of the areola
- The degree of breast sagging
- Skin quality and skin elasticity as well as the amount of extra skin

There are many variations to the procedure, however one of the most common is a pattern with three incisions:

- Around the areola
- Vertically down from the areola to the breast crease
- Horizontally along the breast crease

Through these incisions, the underlying breast tissue is lifted and reshaped to improve breast contour and firmness. The nipple and areola are repositioned to a natural, more youthful height. If necessary, enlarged areolas are reduced by excising skin at the perimeter. Excess breast skin is removed to compensate for a loss of elasticity.

Alternative techniques eliminate either the horizontal incision at the breast crease, the vertical incision from the areola to the breast crease, or sometimes both. In any case, incisions are usually placed so that they can be hidden under clothing and swimsuits. Nonremovable sutures are layered deep within the breast tissue to create and support the newly shaped breasts. Sutures, skin adhesives and/or surgical tape may be used to close the skin.

---

* Les Bolton, MD, FACS, of the Cosmetic Surgery Specialists Group of Beverly Hills, Clinical Instructor of Plastic Surgery, USC School of Medicine and Diplomate of the American Board of Plastic Surgery, contributed to this section.

# BREAST LIFT

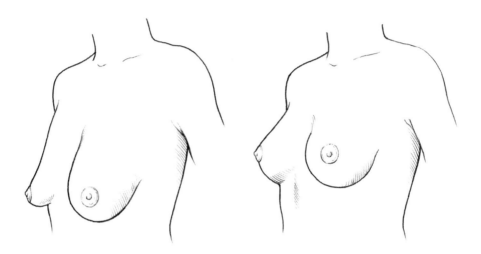

**Doctor: indicate incision location**
**Doctor: identify new location of nipple**

# Breast Lift Checklist

✔ What does this operation accomplish?

_____

_____

✔ What type of anesthesia is used?

_____

_____

✔ How long does the operation last?

_____

_____

✔ Is the operation done in the hospital?

_____

_____

✔ How long will I be off work? When may I resume exercise?

_____

_____

✔ What if unsightly scars form?

_____

_____

✔ What happens if I become pregnant?

_____

_____

✔ Will I lose feeling in the nipples?

_____

_____

✔ Are implants also needed?

_____

_____

✔ How long does the breast lift last?

_____

_____

✔ How painful is this procedure? How will the pain be controlled?

_____

_____

✔ On average, how many of these procedures do you perform annually?

_____

_____

✔ For this procedure, what percentage of your patients require a "touch-up" or "redo"?

_____

_____

# Notes:

_Modern medicine is a gift, but no amount of surgery is going to give any of us the body we had when we were kids._

**— Susan Gail**
**"Body Contouring in the United States"**
_Cosmetic Surgery Times,_ **September 2001**

# BREAST REDUCTION*
## *(Reduction Mammaplasty)*

Breast reduction is more commonly performed through incisions with surgical removal of the excess fat, glandular tissue and skin that contribute to large, pendulous breasts. The most common approach is a keyhole incision pattern.

The nipple, which remains tethered to its original blood and nerve supply, is then repositioned. The areola is reduced by excising skin at the perimeter, if necessary. The vertical incisions are brought together to reshape the now smaller breast. Nonremovable sutures are layered deep within the breast tissue to create and support the newly shaped breasts; sutures, skin adhesive and/or surgical tape close the skin.

There are alternative incision patterns that may be recommended depending on the amount of tissue and skin to be removed and the quality of skin elasticity. One is a circular pattern around the areola. Another is a racket-shaped pattern with an incision around the areola and vertically down to the breast crease. Occasionally, for extremely large pendulous breasts, the nipple and areola may need to be removed and transplanted to a higher position on the breast. In any case, the incision lines that remain are visible and permanent, although usually well concealed beneath a swimsuit or bra.

In some cases, excess fat may be removed through liposuction in conjunction with excision techniques. If breast size is largely due to fatty tissue and excess skin is not a factor, liposuction alone may be used for breast reduction. In every case, the technique used to reduce the size of breasts is determined by individual conditions, breast composition, amount of reduction desired, and patient and surgeon preference.

---

*   Les Bolton, MD, FACS, of the Cosmetic Surgery Specialists Group of Beverly Hills, Clinical Instructor of Plastic Surgery, USC School of Medicine and Diplomate of the American Board of Plastic Surgery, contributed to this section.

# BREAST REDUCTION

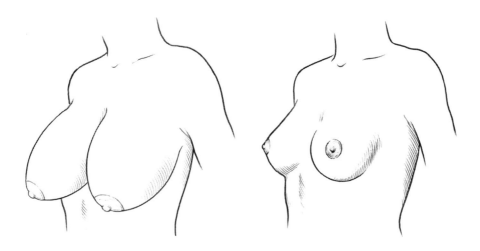

**Doctor: indicate incision location**
**Doctor: identify new location of nipple**

# Breast Reduction Checklist

✔ Will breast reduction influence my ability to breast-feed?

_____

_____

✔ Can anything be done if I am disappointed in my breasts' shape or size after surgery?

_____

_____

✔ What if my nipples are not at the same level, or point differently after surgery? Can this be fixed?

_____

_____

✔ If I develop thick unsightly scars, how can they be improved?

_____

_____

✔ What are my options if my nipple must be grafted and could potentially die? What can be done?

_____

_____

✔ My friend had to get a mammogram before breast reduction surgery. Why?

_____

_____

✔ I was advised to get "liposuction of the armpit" at the same time as my breast reduction. Can you explain why?

_____

_____

✔ What are the chances I will need a blood transfusion? Can I donate my own blood ahead of time?

_____

_____

✔ How long must I wait for the swelling to go down to see the final
result?

_____

_____

✔ What type of anesthesia is used?

_____

_____

✔ Where is the operation performed? What factors would mandate
hospital-level care?

_____

_____

✔ Is there a way of reducing the breast without the traditional breast
reduction scars?

_____

_____

✔ How long does the operation last?

_____

_____

✔ How long will I be off work?

_____

_____

✔ When may I return to full exercise?

_____

_____

✔ What if I become pregnant? Will I lose feeling in the nipples?

_____

_____

✔ Does breast reduction increase the risk of breast cancer?

_____

_____

✔ Do you believe my reduction will qualify for insurance coverage,
and will your office assist me with precertification?

_____

_____

✔ How painful is this procedure?  How will the pain be controlled?

_____

_____

✔ On average, how many of these procedures do you perform annually?

_____

_____

✔ For this procedure, what percentage of your patients require a "touch-up" or "redo"?

_____

_____

# Notes:

_____

Aesthetic surgeons can feel pressured by patient demands, even unrealistic ones.

**— Stanley A. Klatsky, MD**
**Editor in Chief of *Aesthetic Surgery Journal***
**"Surgical Marathons: Is Marketing Hype Dictating Practice Standards?"**
***Aesthetic Surgery Journal* May/June 2004**

# LIPOSUCTION*
## (Lipoplasty)

Liposuction removes unwanted fat deposits from specific areas of the body, including upper arms, chest, abdomen, buttocks, hips, thighs, knees, calves and ankles. *Liposuction is not a substitute for legitimate weight reduction programs* but rather a method of removing localized fat that won't respond to dieting and exercise.  Since the newly formed contour is dependent on contraction of the overlying skin, the best candidates for liposuction are those patients who are young with good skin quality and not obese.

---

*    Les Bolton, MD, FACS, of the Cosmetic Surgery Specialists Group of Beverly Hills, Clinical Instructor of Plastic Surgery, USC School of Medicine and Diplomate of the American Board of Plastic Surgery, contributed to this section.

# LIPOSUCTION

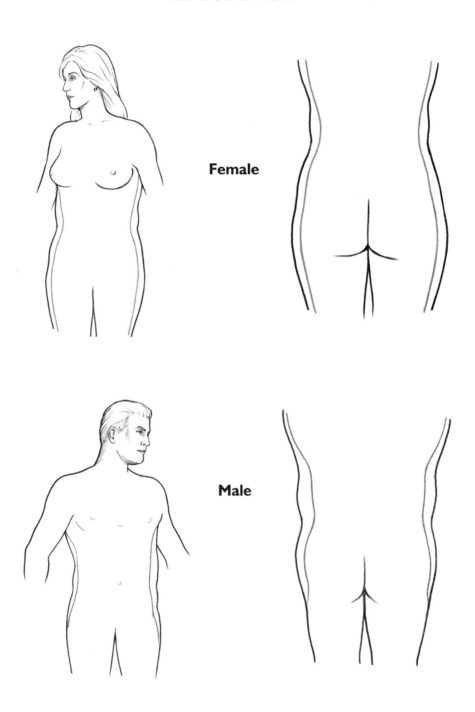

**Female**

**Male**

**Doctor: indicate incision location**

# Liposuction Checklist

✔ Is there an age limit for liposuction?
_____
_____

✔ Are certain areas of the body where skin elasticity is poor less
satisfactory for liposuction?
_____
_____

✔ If major liposuction is performed, will I need a blood transfusion?
Should I "bank" my own blood?
_____
_____

✔ Should large-volume liposuction be done in the hospital?
_____
_____

✔ My skin forms keloid scars. How big an issue is this for liposuction?
_____
_____

✔ Should I expect dimpling of the skin after liposuction?
_____
_____

✔ If one gains weight after liposuction, what happens to the
previously liposuctioned areas? Will the areas that have not been
treated tend to show greater evidence of weight gain? Will I look
strange?
_____
_____

✔ Can an area be liposuctioned more than once?
_____
_____

✔ How long will I be off work? How long does bruising last?

_____
_____

✔ How painful is this procedure?  How will the pain be controlled?

_____
_____

✔ When can I return to exercise?

_____
_____

✔ What type of anesthesia is used?

_____
_____

✔ How much fat can be removed?

_____
_____

✔ What parts of the body can be suctioned?

_____
_____

✔ Can liposuction be done at the same time as other procedures?

_____
_____

✔ If I am now losing weight, should I delay having liposuction?

_____
_____

✔ What happens if I gain weight later?

_____
_____

✔ How is liposuction done?

_____
_____

✔ Will liposuction remove cellulite?

_____

_____

✔ Will things such as dents and ripples occur after liposuction? If so, how are they corrected?

_____

_____

✔ On average, how many of these procedures do you perform annually?

_____

_____

✔ For this procedure, what percentage of your patients require a "touch-up" or "redo"?

_____

_____

We know that longer surgeries inevitably carry greater risk.

**— Stanley A. Klatsky, MD**
**Editor in Chief of _Aesthetic Surgery Journal_**
**"Surgical Marathons: Is Marketing Hype Dictating Practice Standards?"**
**— _Aesthetic Surgery Journal_ May/June 2004**

# Notes:

_In aesthetic surgical procedures, including lipoplasty, the proper emphasis should be on a patient's safety._

**— Discussion by Robert Singer, MD**
**Practice Advisor on Liposuction Plastic Surgery**

# TUMMY TUCK*
## (Abdominoplasty)

This procedure, classified as major cosmetic surgery, removes excess skin and fat from the mid and lower abdomen. Abdominal muscles also may be tightened as part of the procedure. The objective of this surgery is to correct a protruding abdomen caused by pregnancy or genetic predisposition. The degree of surgery is dependent on the amount of excess tissue in place; therefore, patients who intend to lose (a significant amount of) weight should postpone surgery. Likewise, women planning future pregnancies may want to defer the procedure, particularly when seeking to tighten their abdominals. These could separate during the "stretching" process of pregnancy. The appearance of existing abdominal scars may worsen.

A tummy tuck is individualized to your specific condition and may involve:

- Excess localized fat in the abdominal area
- Loose and sagging skin in the abdominal region
- Weakened or separated abdominal muscles due to pregnancy, weight loss and/or aging

One or all of these conditions may be present and can be surgically improved by a tummy tuck. A tummy tuck cannot correct stretch marks, although these may be removed or somewhat improved if they are primarily located on the areas where excess skin will be excised, generally those treated areas below the belly button.

Surgical removal of excess fat and skin may be combined with liposuction during a tummy tuck. There are variations to tummy tuck surgery; the technique selected is dependent on the degree of correction necessary to achieve a flatter profile and firmer abdomen. Incision length

---

* Les Bolton, MD, FACS, of the Cosmetic Surgery Specialists Group of Beverly Hills, Clinical Instructor of Plastic Surgery, USC School of Medicine and Diplomate of the American Board of Plastic Surgery, contributed to this section.

and pattern depend on the amount and location of excess skin to be removed, as well as personal preference and surgical judgment.

Liposuction may be used in conjunction with a tummy tuck or to recontour other areas of the body by removing localized excess fat deposits. Other body contouring procedures may be performed separately or in the same surgical session as a tummy tuck. However, not all patients are good candidates for combined procedures. Your case will be evaluated on an individual basis.

# TUMMY TUCK

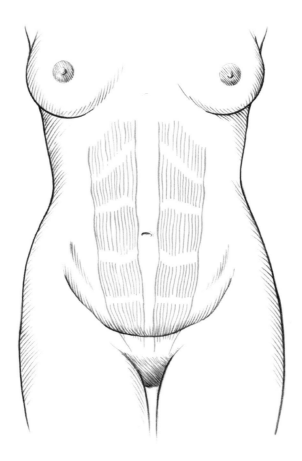

**Doctor: indicate incision location**

# Tummy Tuck Checklist

✔ What factors determine if correction of my abdominal fullness can be accomplished by liposuction vs. a tummy tuck?

_____

_____

✔ What is a "partial" or "mini-tummy tuck"? Am I a candidate?

_____

_____

✔ What happens if I gain weight afterward? Lose weight?

_____

_____

✔ Can problems occur if I become pregnant after surgery?

_____

_____

✔ Will there be obvious scars?

_____

_____

✔ What are the chances of keloid scars?

_____

_____

✔ I do a strenuous workout program including sit-ups. How long before I can resume these activities?

_____

_____

✔ What is the most common complication? How is it corrected?

_____

_____

✔ What is the most serious complication? How is this handled?

_____

_____

✔ How long will I be off work? When may I resume full exercise?

_____

_____

✔ How long does the operation take?

_____

_____

✔ Where is the operation performed?

_____

_____

✔ What type of anesthesia is used?

_____

_____

✔ What about the endoscopic tummy tuck?

_____

_____

✔ Will there be scars?

_____

_____

✔ What if I become pregnant afterward?

_____

_____

✔ How painful is this procedure?  How will the pain be controlled?

_____

_____

✔ On average, how many of these procedures do you perform annually?

_____

_____

✔ For this procedure, what percentage of your patients require a "touch-up" or "redo"?

_____

_____

# Notes:

_____
_____
_____
_____
_____
_____
_____
_____
_____
_____
_____
_____
_____
_____
_____
_____
_____
_____
_____
_____
_____
_____
_____
_____
_____
_____
_____

The Rodeo Drive belly button: tummy tuck used to be purely debulking and damage control. Forty or 50 years ago, sometimes the belly button was just removed. We've changed the technique slightly — it actually creates a somewhat better hood at the top, for piercing, and throws a bit of a deeper shadow, so it looks more natural in a bikini and low-rider jeans.

**— Lloyd Krieger, MD**
**in "Glimpses,"** _University of Chicago Magazine_**, December 2004**
**Courtesy A.N. Epstein, BA, MBA**

# FACE AND NECK PROCEDURES

~

## CHEEK IMPLANTS
### (Malarplasty)

Some men and women, to improve and achieve facial structure, benefit from "cheek implants." Cheek implantation is analogous to chin implantation. Solid, silicone-plastic, FDA-approved, preformed "parts" are placed onto the existing cheekbones, beneath the skin's surface, to give more satisfactory prominence to the cheek areas.

# CHEEK IMPLANT

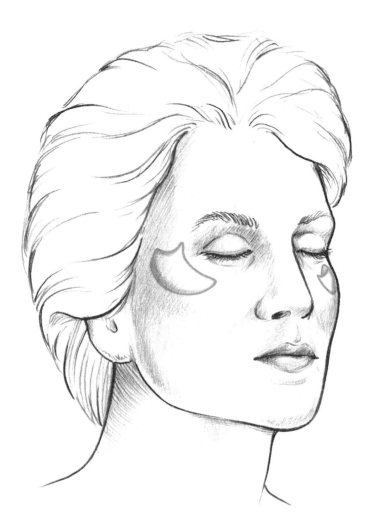

**Doctor: indicate incision location**

# Cheek Implant Checklist:

✔ May I see the implant you suggest?

_____

_____

✔ Why do you recommend this particular style, shape and size for me?

_____

_____

✔ What is the chance of "slippage" or rejection? Will this cause damage to my tissues?

_____

_____

✔ What route of insertion do you recommend? Why?

_____

_____

✔ If the cheek implants are inserted through the mouth, is there a greater chance of infection?

_____

_____

✔ If inserted via a lower-eyelid incision, can the eyelids be injured or malformed by the implant surgery?

_____

_____

✔ How are implants anchored or kept in place?

_____

_____

✔ Will there by numbness of the face and/or lips? If so, for how long?

_____

_____

✔ If one or both of the implants ever have to be removed, when can they be replaced?

_____
_____

✔ If I choose not to have the implants replaced, how will I look?

_____
_____

✔ How painful is this procedure? How will the pain be controlled?

_____
_____

✔ On average, how many of these procedures do you perform annually?

_____
_____

✔ For this procedure, what percentage of your patients require a "touch-up" or "redo"?

_____
_____

# Notes:

_____

_____

_____

_____

_____

_____

_____

_____

_____

_____

_____

_____

_____

_____

_____

_____

_____

_____

_____

_____

_____

_____

_____

_____

_____

_____

_____

_____

_____

If you decide that you want to have surgery to change something about yourself, make sure that you do your research and find a doctor who won't change you into somebody even you won't recognize. Rather, choose a surgeon who helps you find a look that fits you as an individual!

— *The Look,*
**Celebrity Makeup Artist Bobbe Joy**
*Women on Top,* **2004**

# CHIN AUGMENTATION
## (Mentoplasty)

Correction of a receding chin is frequently performed simultaneously with face and neck lifting, neck sculpturing or nasal cosmetic surgery. Today's techniques utilize plastic inserts that are quite safe and not likely to dislodge. They may be inserted through the mouth or through a fine incision hidden under the chin (discussed later in Face & Neck Lifting). The latter technique is preferred by most surgeons.

# CHIN AUGMENTATION

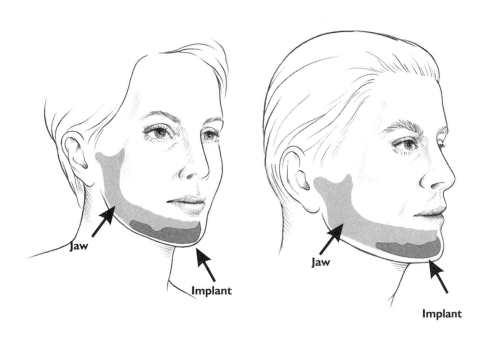

**Female**                    **Male**

**Doctor: indicate the incision location
(inside mouth or under chin)**

# Chin Augmentation Checklist

✔ What kind of implant material is used to build up the chin?

_____
_____

✔ Is it safe? Is it FDA approved? Can I see one?

_____
_____

✔ How long has this type of implant been used?

_____
_____

✔ How are they inserted?

_____
_____

✔ What is the chance of rejection? If the implant is being rejected, how is it managed? Will this cause damage to my tissues?

_____
_____

✔ What are the chances of infection? What if this happens to me?

_____
_____

✔ Is there a possibility the implant can shift position? If this happens, what do we do? If the implant has to be removed for any reason, can it be replaced later? How long an interval must I wait? How will I look while waiting for replacement?

_____
_____

✔ How painful is this procedure? How will the pain be controlled?

_____
_____

✔ On average, how many of these procedures do you perform annually?

_____

_____

✔ For this procedure, what percentage of your patients require a "touch-up" or "redo"?

_____

_____

# Notes:

_You have to know **what you are doing and what the patient wants.**
Patients are experts on their own faces._

— **Edward O. Terino, MD**
**_Cosmetic Surgery Times,_** **March 2005**

# CORRECTION OF PROTRUDING EARS
## (*Otoplasty*)

Ear position can be corrected on adults or on children five years or older. The objective of the surgery is to permanently recontour the pliable ear cartilage. This is done by sculpting and reshaping the cartilage through incisions hidden on the back surface of the ear.

Repositioning protruding ears is the most common form of ear surgery performed. It is widely performed with a good record of safety and fulfillment of patient goals. Even when only one ear appears to protrude, ear surgery may be performed on both ears to achieve a more balanced result. Just as all of our faces are asymmetric to some degree, results of ear surgery may not be completely symmetric. However, the goal is to create an ear as normal as possible in structure and proportional balance relative to other facial features.

Ear surgery revision is sometimes requested by adults who are dissatisfied with a prior surgery. This may include an unnatural appearance, overcorrection, in which ears appear to be sharply "pinned" back, and irregularities of the ear folds. Concern with residual earlobe prominence is also common.

# EAR SURGERY

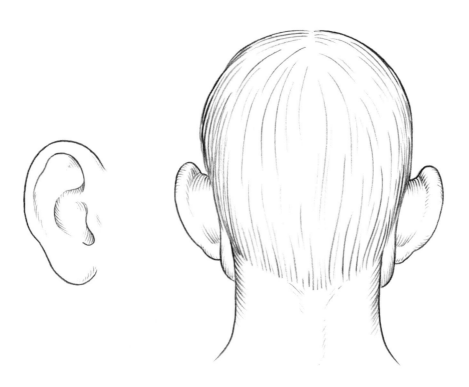

**Doctor: indicate incision location**

# Correction of Protruding Ears Checklist

✔ Is there a difference between a child's and an adult's operation?
_____
_____

✔ What will keep my ears closer to my head? Will they "pull out" after a period of time?
_____
_____

✔ One ear is different from the other. Can they be made exactly the same?
_____
_____

✔ How bad is the swelling? When do you think I can appear in public without any dressing?
_____
_____

✔ Will the operation have any effect on my hearing?
_____
_____

✔ I have big earlobes. Can they be made smaller?
_____
_____

✔ I understand the ears are "numb" for a time after surgery. Can you explain why and how long this numbness will last?
_____
_____

✔ What will the dressing look like? How long is it worn?
_____
_____

✔ Are the stitches dissolvable or do they require removal? If the latter, how long after surgery are they removed?

_____

_____

✔ Will I need to wear a ski or headband for some time after the surgery?

_____

_____

✔ What kind of anesthesia is used?

_____

_____

✔ How painful is this procedure? How will the pain be controlled?

_____

_____

✔ On average, how many of these procedures do you perform annually?

_____

_____

✔ For this procedure, what percentage of your patients require a "touch-up" or "redo"?

_____

_____

# Notes:

_____
_____
_____
_____
_____
_____
_____
_____
_____
_____
_____
_____
_____
_____
_____
_____
_____
_____
_____
_____
_____
_____
_____
_____
_____
_____
_____
_____
_____
_____
_____
_____

# EYELID SURGERY
## (Blepharoplasty)

The objective of upper eyelid surgery is to remove the fold of the skin that forms between the eyelash and eyebrow, which conceals the natural eyelid and obscures the cleft that separates the lid from the brow. Eyes appear "hooded." This profound pleat-like fold of skin may interfere with normal vision when it becomes heavy.

Standard upper lid surgery removes this excess skin and fatty tissue through an incision neatly placed in that natural crease between the eyelid and eyebrow.

Lower eyelid surgery is performed primarily to remove "bags" caused by bulging fatty tissue beneath the skin. Upper and lower eyelid cosmetic surgery can be performed independently of each other or together.

# EYE SURGERY

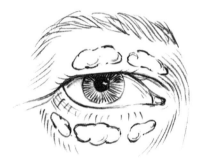 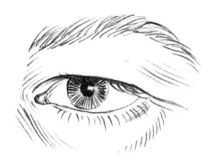

**Doctor: indicate incision location**

# Upper Eyelid Surgery Checklist

✔ Does the eyebrow have to be lifted with every upper eyelid surgery?

_____

_____

✔ Is eyelid and/or forehead-brow surgery part of facelift procedure?

_____

_____

✔ I am of Asian decent. Is the procedure for eyelid surgery different?

_____

_____

✔ I've heard that some people have trouble closing their eyes after upper eyelid surgery. Why does this happen? How is it corrected? Will this happen to me?

_____

_____

✔ My upper eyelids are so heavy that my vision is impaired. This being the case, does my operation qualify for insurance benefits? What steps must we take to have my insurance company approve the procedure?

_____

_____

✔ I have dry eye. Will surgery impact that condition? If so, can anything be done in advance to minimize potential effects?

_____

_____

✔ What are the advantages and disadvantages of laser vs. traditional surgery?

_____

_____

✔ How soon can I wear my contact lenses after upper eyelid surgery?

_____

_____

✔ On average, how many of these procedures do you perform annually?

_____

_____

✔ For this procedure, what percentage of your patients require a "touch-up" or "redo"?

_____

_____

# Lower Eyelid Surgery Checklist

✔ I have extra skin and "puffiness" under my eyes. How are each of these problems managed?

_____

_____

✔ What precautions are taken to prevent that pulled-down, hound-dog look?

_____

_____

✔ Is my anatomy such that I need to have the fat re-positioned rather than removed? Might I need an implant or filling material?

_____

_____

✔ If I have wrinkled skin, how is that usually treated?

_____

_____

✔ Can eyelid surgery eliminate the dark color?

_____

_____

✔ Laser surgery. How does it differ from traditional surgery? What are the advantages and disadvantages of both?

_____

_____

✔ Based upon my appearance, am I a candidate for the external or
internal incisions?

_____

_____

✔ Depending on incision location, what kind of stitches are used and
how long are they in place?

_____

_____

✔ How painful is this procedure? How will the pain be controlled?

_____

_____

✔ On average, how many of these procedures do you perform
annually?

_____

_____

✔ For this procedure, what percentage of your patients require a
"touch-up" or "redo"?

_____

_____

# Notes:

_____
_____
_____
_____
_____
_____
_____
_____
_____
_____
_____
_____
_____
_____
_____
_____
_____
_____
_____
_____
_____
_____
_____
_____
_____
_____
_____
_____

## Beauty Is More Than Skin Deep

A plastic surgeon does not simply alter a man's face. He alters the man's inner self. The incisions he makes are more than skin deep. They frequently cut deep into the psyche as well. I decided a long time ago that this is an awesome responsibility and that I owe it to my patients and to myself to know something about what I am doing. No responsible MD would attempt to perform extensive plastic surgery without specialized knowledge and training. Just so, I feel that if changing a man's face is going to change the inner man as well, I have a responsibility to acquire specialized knowledge in that field, also.

**— Maxwell Maltz, MD, FICS**
*Psycho-Cybernetics, a New*
*Way to Get More Living out of Life*

# FACE & NECK LIFT
## (Cervicofacial Rhytidectomy)

Face and neck lifting offer several alternatives, because you are dealing with multiple components. Common procedures include tightening under the chin or about the neck, sculpting the jawline and cheeks, or removal of jowls.

# FACE & NECK LIFT

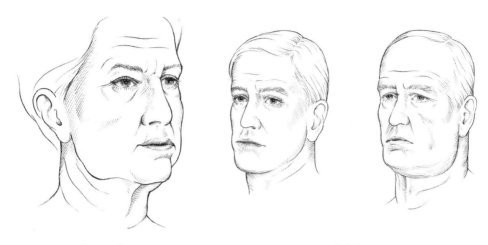

**Female**                                            **Male**

**Doctor: indicate incision location;
boundaries of surgery, area of dissection**

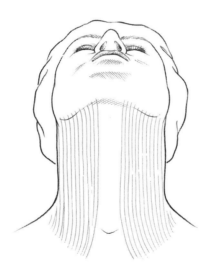

**Doctor: indicate management of neck muscle**

# Face & Neck Lift Checklist

✔ Do you do that "deep plane" facelift? Is it appropriate for me? If you do not do "deep plane," how do you lift the sagging facial tissue? Will skin be removed?

_____

_____

✔ How will the neck be managed? Is there a separate neck incision? Where? Does the sagging platysma muscle need attention?

_____

_____

✔ Do you place suction drains? If so, why? For how long? Where do they exit? How are they removed? Is it painful?

_____

_____

✔ If drains are not employed, is tissue sealant, a glue-like substance, used?

_____

_____

✔ How long do you expect the facelift procedure to last? What factors might cause less longevity? Is the second procedure as extensive? How might it be different? I've seen people who look like they "walked behind a jet engine." The face had a "pulled" look. What is the reason for that? Can you assure me that I will not have a similar result?

_____

_____

✔ Does every facelift include eyelid surgery and/or forehead and eyebrow lifting? Does every facelift include the neck?

_____

_____

✔ Why do some mature people have a "nose job" with their facelift? Is this done routinely? Is it right for me?

_____

_____

✔ I've heard that some people have a chin implant placed at the time of facelifting. Would I need to have one?

_____

_____

✔ Am I too old for a full facelift? Is there an age limit?

_____

_____

✔ Will I lose my facial expression?

_____

_____

✔ Does a facelift correct laugh lines around the mouth, or frown lines in the forehead and between the eyes? Will it remove the grooves that run between my nose and the outer corner of my mouth?

_____

_____

✔ Will my hair be shaved off? When can I wash my hair? When can I color my hair?

_____

_____

✔ I'm a man. Where will the incisions be placed? Will they show? Will my beard-line shift?

_____

_____

✔ How painful is this procedure? How will the pain be controlled?

_____

_____

✔ On average, how many of these procedures do you perform annually?

_____

_____

✔ For this procedure, what percentage of your patients require a "touch-up" or "redo"?

_____

_____

In 1919 Dr. Adalbert G. Bettman introduced the extensive facelift incision that is still the basis of today's procedures.

— **Ellen Feldman**
**"Before and After"**
*American Heritage*, **February/March 2004**

# Notes:

_Radical facelift procedures, such as midface lifts and deep-plain or composite facelifts, increase the potential for complications and increase morbidity. Although a small percentage of patients may require these radical techniques to achieve optimal results, there is no evidence that radical procedures produce better or longer-lasting improvements in the vast majority of patients than do properly performed standard methods._

**— Simon Fredericks, MD**
**"Radical Facelift Surgery: A Plea for Caution"**
_Aesthetic Surgery Journal,_ **January/February 2002**

# FACIAL REJUVENATION: LASER OR CHEMICAL
## (Nonsurgical Wrinkle Removal)

The aim of both processes is to destroy the outermost skin layers and thereby induce Nature to replace the older, wrinkled, sun-damaged skin with new, smooth, unwrinkled skin, free of age spots and other precancerous areas that are the hallmark of aged skin. The technical difference between laser and chemical peel treatments is how the outer layers of skin are destroyed. Lasers use a high-intensity, invisible beam of light energy that destroys superficial skin cells by boiling the water inside the cells. The treatment's strength is a function of intensity and length of time the beam is allowed to strike the skin. Lower power and shorter exposure time translates to less skin destruction and a shorter healing time, but a less profound result. Conversely, the deeper the damage to the skin, the more exuberant the healing process that generates the smoothest, tightest, most wrinkle-free new skin. Chemical peels achieve their result by a controlled chemical burn that instigates the repair process. The spectrum of peeling agents or acids includes salicylic acid (a cousin of aspirin) at the weak end, and trichloroacetic acid (TCA) or phenol (carbolic acid) at the strong end. Phenol is considered by most sophisticated practitioners the most consistent, predictable and effective peeling agent. It is the agent preferred for deep peeling and creates the most impressive rejuvenation result.

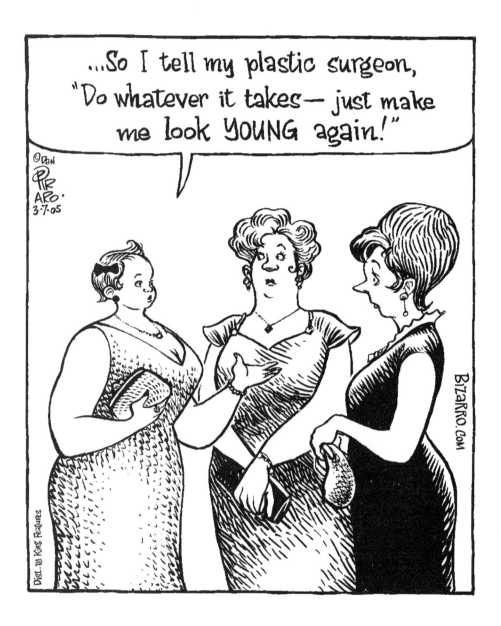

# Facial Rejuvenation Checklist

✔ What is the difference between a chemical peel and a laser peel?
_____
_____

✔ Which is better for me?
_____
_____

✔ Is it true that not everyone is a satisfactory candidate for this procedure?
_____
_____

✔ How do I know if I am a good candidate? Is there a test to see if my skin is appropriate?
_____
_____

✔ Is there any special skin preparation necessary? Are there any products or medications I should not be placing on my face prior to the procedure?
_____
_____

✔ Is it better to have the procedure done at a relatively young age, such as the 40s ? Or should I wait until the wrinkles are "really bad," in the 60s or 70s?
_____
_____

✔ What about my wrinkled neck? Can it be peeled or lasered too?
_____
_____

✔ Can facial and/or neck surgery be done at the same time as chemical peeling or laser?
_____
_____

✔ Are all parts of the face treated? What are the pros and cons of treating the whole face vs. sections of the face?
_____
_____

✔ Can blotchiness occur? If so, what can be done?

_____

_____

✔ Is it true you can never go back into the sun after this procedure?

_____

_____

✔ Will resurfacing the skin cause permanent lightening of my natural color?

_____

_____

✔ What will I look like during recovery?

_____

_____

✔ When can I wear makeup again?

_____

_____

✔ How long do these procedures last? Is it true that smoking, drinking and other poor health habits will shorten the improvement's life span?

_____

_____

✔ How painful is this procedure? How will the pain be controlled?

_____

_____

✔ On average, how many of these procedures do you perform annually?

_____

_____

✔ For this procedure, what percentage of your patients require a "touch-up" or "redo"?

_____

_____

# Notes:

_In the same year I bought a new car and had a chemical skin peel. Twenty years later, my face is still smooth, but I'm on my fourth car._

**— Barbara V., patient**

# FOREHEAD & EYEBROW LIFT
## (Browplasty)

As men and women age, their eyebrows may droop, creating a somewhat sad or oppressed look. Such sagging may coexist or be independent of other signs of facial aging. Correction of the forehead and brow may be done concurrently with any of the other surgical procedures.

Forehead/brow lifting yields a more natural, brighter appearance by elevating and tightening the eyebrows, forehead skin and muscles. In certain instances, frown lines and forehead creases also mildly improve. Results are best when brows are elevated to a "natural" level. Overdoing this procedure will create a very unsatisfactory "always surprised" look. This result should be avoided, since it cannot be easily corrected.

Your brow lift will be individualized according to factors such as your skin, muscle tone, forehead height and bone structure, taking into consideration the specific conditions you wish to correct. Although incisions are typically concealed within hair-bearing scalp, patients who have thinning hair or are bald may still benefit from a brow lift. All of these individual factors will be considered when determining the appropriate technique or combination of procedures to best achieve your realistic goals.

A brow lift is a surgical procedure; nonsurgical rejuvenation treatments will not achieve the same results, though in some instances they may help delay the time for which a brow lift is appropriate. Brow lift incisions typically are closed with removable sutures, skin adhesives, surgical tape or special clips. Brow elevation may be maintained by the use of permanent sutures, small surgical screws, or an absorbable fixation device placed inconspicuously at the temples.

A brow lift may take two hours or more, depending on the extent of rejuvenation, the techniques used and any additional procedures performed at the same time. Rejuvenation procedures typically performed in conjunction with a brow lift include eyelid surgery to rejuvenate aging eyes and a facelift to correct aging changes in the mid to lower face and neck regions.

# BROW LIFT

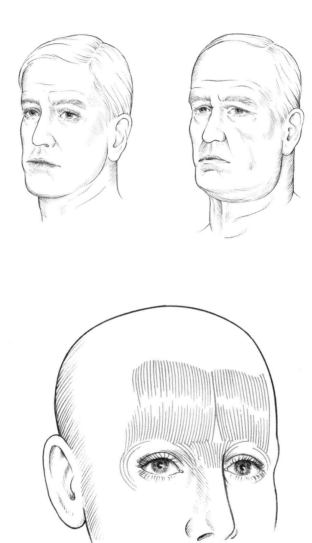

**Doctor: indicate incision location(s)**

# Forehead & Eyebrow Lifting Checklist

✔ What is the difference between "endoscopic" forehead brow lift and older coronal techniques? Describe the "older" procedure. Is the newer one better? With the "endoscopic" technique, where are the incisions made?

_____

_____

✔ Can the brows be lifted via the eyelid incisions?

_____

_____

✔ My biggest problems are the deep lines between my eyes from frowning. Will forehead or eyebrow lifting help this?

_____

_____

✔ My brows hang so low that they seem to cause problems with my vision. Does this mean both the brows and eyelids must be lifted?

_____

_____

✔ Is there a chance the nerves to the forehead muscles can be injured? If so, what will I look like? Can this be repaired?

_____

_____

✔ Will there be a lot of bruising around the eyes and forehead?

_____

_____

✔ How soon can I return to work and normal activities?

_____

_____

✔ How painful is this procedure? How will the pain be controlled?

_____

_____

✔ On average, how many of these procedures do you perform annually?

_____

_____

✔ For this procedure, what percentage of your patients require a "touch-up" or "redo"?

_____

_____

# Notes:

_____
_____
_____
_____
_____
_____
_____
_____
_____
_____
_____
_____
_____
_____
_____
_____
_____
_____
_____
_____
_____
_____
_____
_____
_____
_____
_____
_____
_____
_____
_____

_You can argue the merits philosophically, but the reality is that when we look at other people, we tend to make superficial judgments based on attractiveness or unattractiveness of facial features. Better-looking people fare better in life._

**— Robert Kotler, MD, FACS**
**_Cosmetic Surgery Times_, September 2001**

# NASAL SURGERY
## (Rhinoplasty)

Nasal cosmetic surgery is still the most frequently performed cosmetic procedure. It is also the most complex and sophisticated of all the cosmetic surgeries. Often, the surgeon is also called upon to improve breathing. Unfortunately, today, due to deterioration in some training programs, surgeons are graduating from residency training programs ill-suited by lack of experience and specific training to be satisfactory nasal cosmetic surgeons. This is a procedure for which you want to select the right surgeon, because the first surgical visit to the nose is the easiest. Re-dos are very tough. Thus, you want to do it right—the first time.

---

While facelifts and breast augmentation were on the rise in postwar America, rhinoplasty, the earliest plastic procedure, remained the most popular operation. From the end of World War I until our current era of medical tourism, which sends patients hurrying around the world in search of good treatment at the right place with the best views, cosmetic surgery was a particularly American specialty, and the "nose job" was the typical American procedure.

— **Ellen Feldman**
**"Before and After"**
*American Heritage*, **February/ March 2004**

---

Dear Dr. Kotler,

It has been a month now since I had my surgery and I wanted to write to you to thank you and let you know how much I appreciate everything you have done for me.

I am satisfied with the decision we made and could not be happier with the results. More importantly than the cosmetic reason, the functional improvement was amazing. Because of my severe allergies, prior to my surgery I was taking antihistamines every day with no relief. As a result of my nasal surgery, I no longer have difficulty breathing and the daily allergies I suffered from are gone. As an internist I will be sure to recommend this procedure for my patients suffering from the same problem.

— **Richard Roman, MD**

# NASAL SURGERY

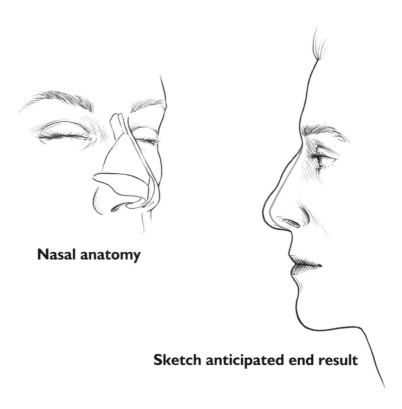

**Nasal anatomy**

**Sketch anticipated end result**

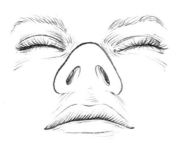

**Doctor: indicate incision location if external
or "open" technique is used.**

# Nasal Surgery Checklist

✔ What parts of my nose need attention? Describe my new nose.
_____
_____

✔ Can you assure me that the nose will look natural? Why do some "nose jobs" look unnatural?
_____
_____

✔ Will you have to break my nose?
_____
_____

✔ Will I have incisions hidden within my nose, or an external incision between nostrils? Why?
_____
_____

✔ Does my nose require the insertion of an artificial plastic part, or bone or cartilage taken from the inside of the nose, or even from the ear, rib or other distant body location?
_____
_____

✔ When I smile, my nose comes down and nearly meets my lip. Can that be corrected? How? Will it affect my lip?
_____
_____

✔ What is the earliest age at which cosmetic nasal surgery can be performed?
_____
_____

✔ Is it true that the nose grows as people get older? What can be done about that?
_____
_____

✔ Can I combine nasal surgery with other cosmetic facial surgery?
_____
_____

✔ I want to have my breathing improved at the same time. Can this be done? My health insurance will cover the breathing portion of the operation. Does having cosmetic surgery at the same time present a problem to my insurance company?

_____

_____

✔ If I have both cosmetic and breathing surgery, what is the difference in recovery time?

_____

_____

✔ How long will the internal packing be in place?

_____

_____

✔ How long before the swelling goes down and I look decent?

_____

_____

✔ When can I resume normal activities? Apply makeup?

_____

_____

✔ Can a too-small nose be made larger?

_____

_____

✔ I have broken capillaries on my nose? Does that mean I can or cannot have nasal surgery?

_____

_____

✔ How painful is this procedure? How will the pain be controlled?

_____

_____

✔ On average, how many of these procedures do you perform annually?

_____

_____

✔ For this procedure, what percentage of your patients require a "touch-up" or "redo"?

_____

_____

# Notes:

In 1923 Fanny Brice underwent rhinoplasty to transform her nose from what she called "prominent" to "merely decorative," but the aura surrounding the operation, which was performed in her apartment at the Ritz-Carlton in New York City, was more circus like than antiseptic.

— **Ellen Feldman**
**"Before and After"**
*American Heritage*, **February/March 2004**

# Consulting About a Redo?

Be careful! Redos or "revisions" are more technically challenging for any surgeon, even the most specialized and experienced. A perfect result can never be warranted. The decision-making is critical; sometimes, the best decision is to not re-operate. As I advise patients: Better to keep a minor imperfection than to risk a major one.

### Be Sure to Ask About Nonsurgical Options

For some patients, a satisfactory improvement can be obtained without another trip to the operating room. Some "bumps" or "rises" can be permanently flattened by cortisone injections under the skin. Depressions can be permanently filled with liquid medical-grade silicone. An injection of either takes only seconds and can be virtually painless following the application of a topical anesthetic.

There is one nifty and practical way for you to see immediately the obtainable result from a filling injection. The doctor injects sterile saline, under the skin, to plump up the depressed area. This saltwater preparation is a safe, temporary filler that disappears within 20 minutes. We call this a demo or a test drive. If you like what you see, and feel, you may consider opting for this nonsurgical alternative. In addition to avoiding another trip to the OR, there is zero downtime, the cost is far less, and since you are awake — with mirror in hand — you can participate in the "how much will do the job?" decision. Because it is wisest to inject a non-extractable, permanent substance, "little by little," several sessions may be required. But most importantly, you decide when the improved appearance satisfies you. **You're in charge**.

# NECK SCULPTURE
## *(Submentoplasty)*

Neck sculpture optimizes the definition between chin and neck by removing excess fat beneath the skin and, as needed, tightening the sagging platysma neck muscle. Its success is dependent on the neck skin having enough elasticity to retract and redrape satisfactorily after sculpting. Think of a new, tight rubber band, rather than an old, used, stretched-out one.

This procedure is most appropriate for younger patients who have inherited a "double chin" or for those patients who, despite reasonable weight loss, retain a neckline that is still poorly defined. Though not a substitute for the more ambitious face and neck lifting, neck sculpting may indeed delay the day of more extensive procedures, since it addresses the area that is frequently the first to reflect aging.

# NECK SCULPTURE

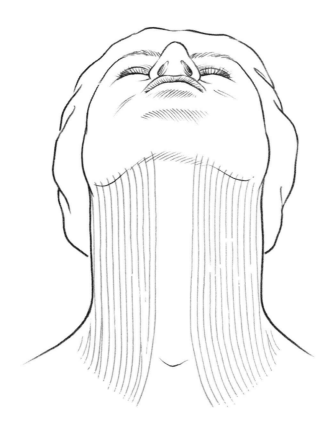

**Doctor: indicate incision location;
boundaries of surgery, area of dissection**

# Neck Sculpture Checklist

✔ Is this the procedure used for a younger person who has a double chin? Should I try diet and exercise first?

_____

_____

✔ What do you actually do in this operation? Do you liposuction to remove fat? Do you tighten muscles?

_____

_____

✔ I am young but have a hanging neck muscle. What can you do about that? Why does elasticity count? If my skin is not taut, is it true that this operation is not appropriate?

_____

_____

✔ How is neck sculpturing different from the neck portion of a face and neck lift?

_____

_____

✔ If I have a chin implant, how does it affect the overall surgery and my recovery?

_____

_____

✔ Are drains put in? For how long? Where do they exit?

_____

_____

✔ How are they removed? Will it be painful?

_____

_____

✔ If drains are not employed, is tissue sealant, a glue-like substance, used?

_____

_____

✔ How soon can I resume normal activities?

_____

_____

✔ What will happen if I gain or lose substantial weight after the procedure is done?

_____

_____

✔ How painful is this procedure? How will the pain be controlled?

_____

_____

✔ On average, how many of these procedures do you perform annually?

_____

_____

✔ For this procedure, what percentage of your patients require a "touch-up" or "redo"?

_____

_____

# Notes:

_____
_____
_____
_____
_____
_____
_____
_____
_____
_____
_____
_____
_____
_____
_____
_____
_____
_____
_____
_____
_____
_____
_____
_____
_____
_____
_____

*A pretty necklace looks better on a beautiful neck.*

**— Arlene Howard**
**Featured patient on**
**E! Entertainment's *Dr. 90210* July 2004**

# 7

# SAFETY FIRST—
# OPERATING ROOM AND
# ANESTHESIA ISSUES:

## *Your Risk Is Not in the Cutting and Sewing*

### Where Will Your Surgeon Operate?

## Hospital

Unless you have a medical condition warranting hospital-level service, or you are a patient under the age of 14 (only hospitals are expected to have medications and equipment suitable for all ages), a hospital may not be your best choice. They are generally large and impersonal. They are expensive, and more importantly, rarely focus on or specialize in cosmetic surgery. Today's hospitals are overtaxed by staff shortages and tight budgets. Their mission is to serve the needs of sick patients. The consequence is that cosmetic surgery patients are rarely treated in an attentive and comforting manner.

## Office Surgical Suites

Assuming they are duly licensed, certified or accredited, and thus meet strict safety and quality-control requirements, doctors' office surgical suites can be adequate and appropriate for cosmetic surgery. Optimally, the facility should be in a medical campus building because it is important to have other doctors available in case of emergency. At the least, there must be a nurse anesthetist or physician-anesthesiologist on the surgical team. Charges for office facilities tend to be far less than those of hospitals, and somewhat less than those of outpatient surgery centers.

## Outpatient Surgery Center

These are appropriate for nearly all cosmetic surgery procedures and are particularly suited for cosmetic procedures. Unlike hospitals, surgery centers offer niche or boutique services that can be exquisitely specialized. Since they typically have two to four operating rooms, there is usually plenty of capable support staff, a critical issue should there be an emergency. Nurses, surgeons and anesthesia specialists are on-site at all times. Surgery centers are best located in buildings devoted to medical services, or on a medical campus. Both provide safe, seasoned, secure places for medical procedures, and professional environments for pre- and post-operation consultations.

Most importantly, surgery centers offer the patient privacy and anonymity in a tranquil, relaxed atmosphere. Fees are typically somewhere between those of a hospital and an office suite outpatient setup.

---

### Operating Facility Checklist:

● Where will the procedure be performed?

✔ A hospital? And if so, as an inpatient (overnight stay) or outpatient (recovery at home or elsewhere)?

_____

_____

✔ An outpatient surgery center?

_____

_____

✔ An office?

_____

_____

### Notes:

_____

_____

_____

_____

_____

_____

_____

_____

_____

● What safety and quality credential(s) does the facility have?

✔ Licensure by the state?

_____

_____

✔ Certification by the U.S. government?

_____

_____

✔ Accreditation Association for Ambulatory Healthcare (**AAAHC**)?

_____

_____

✔ American Association for Accreditation of Ambulatory Surgical Facilities (**AAAASF**)?

_____

_____

✔ Joint Commission on Accreditation of Healthcare Organizations (**JCAHO**)?

_____

_____

## Notes:

_____

_____

_____

_____

_____

_____

_____

_____

_____

_____

_____

If the surgical facility is not a hospital, does it have a transfer agreement with a nearby general hospital? A transfer agreement is a guarantee, for the benefit of the patient, that should hospital-level care be required on an emergency basis, the hospital will automatically and promptly accept the patient for admission. No red tape.

The trend toward office-based and ambulatory center surgery has dramatically increased over the past two decades. Current projections are that by 2005, 80% of all operative procedures will be performed in outpatient facilities. These settings have several potential advantages over hospital-based surgery, including cost containment, personalized attention, convenience, a more flexible schedule, patient privacy, attention to details of patient comfort, a more specialized staff and avoidance of hospital-based infections. Plastic surgery has been at the forefront of this trend.

**— William Mazanitis, MD, and David Miller, MD**
*Anesthesia for Aesthetic Surgery — Plastic Surgery Products, May 2004*

Lloyd Krieger, MBA '92, MD '94, knows that elective plastic surgery patients are different from other surgery cases. They're there to look better, not to get better. "They don't want to come into a hospital with all that implies, he says, "the waiting, the inconvenience, the expense, sitting next to someone waiting for a liver transplant." Enter Krieger's Rodeo Drive Plastic Surgery, the first and only plastic surgery clinic on the glam Beverly Hills shopping strip.

**— "Glimpses"**
*University of Chicago Magazine, December 2004*

# ANESTHESIA: WHO WILL BE "AT THE CONTROLS"?

There are three modes of anesthesia your surgeon will consider:

- Local anesthesia, injected by the surgeon
- Local anesthesia with intravenous sedation
- General anesthesia. The patient is unconscious; vital signs are constantly monitored.

Two different types of medical specialists are qualified to administer anesthesia: Certified Registered Nurse Anesthetists (CRNA) and physician anesthesiologists. Nurse anesthetists officially work under the direction of the surgeon. Nurse anesthetists are licensed registered nurses who have pursued additional specialty training in anesthesia — the nursing parallel of a physician's residency.

Anesthesiologists are medical doctors who have trained in their specialty a minimum of three years after medical school. This specialty is defined as "the practice of internal medicine in the operating and recovery rooms."

You should ask what type of anesthetic the surgeon prefers, whether the administrator of the anesthetic will be a CRNA or an MD (medical doctor) anesthesiologist, and how well the surgeon knows this individual.

If you value the wisdom of selecting a superspecialist cosmetic surgeon, ask that doctor to select an anesthesia specialist who is as specialized as he is. By doing so, you further enhance your prospect of having a safe, comfortable and positive anesthesia experience.

While the chance of a problem with anesthesia is minuscule, if a difficulty should arise, in the wrong hands, it could be catastrophic. You should seek to reduce that risk to the lowest level possible.

## Decide whom you prefer to have administer the anesthetic.

Make your feelings known, without equivocation, to your doctor. It's your body. It's your life.

Whatever the type of anesthesia used, it is essential that the anesthesiologist be experienced in providing anesthesia for aesthetic surgery procedures....

An essential feature of any aesthetic surgery is that the procedure must be performed in the safest way possible.

— **William Mazanitis, MD, and David Miller, MD**
*Anesthesia for Aesthetic Surgery — Plastic Surgery Products,* **May 2004**

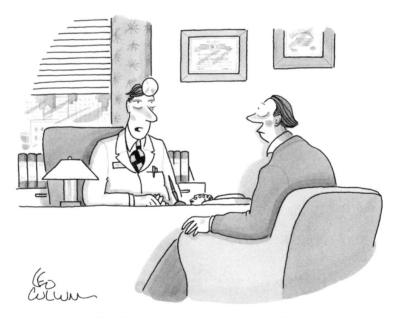

*"You'll be awake during the entire procedure.
The anesthesiologist is on vacation."*

## Anesthesia Checklist:

# What kind of anesthesia?

✔ Will the procedure be performed under *local anesthesia* only (you are completely awake, akin to an office dental procedure)?

_____

_____

✔ If not under local anesthesia, will the procedure be conducted under *local anesthesia with sedation* (conscious sedation; you are very sleepy or asleep but not unconscious) or *general anesthesia*\* (you are unconscious; all vital functions are under the direct control of the anesthesia specialist)?

_____

_____

✔ Who will be responsible for the anesthesia? Who will be at the controls? The surgeon? An RN? A Certified Registered Nurse Anesthetist (CRNA)? An anesthesiologist (MD Specialist, limiting practice to anesthesia)? If an anesthesiologist, is the anesthesiologist certified by the American Board of Anesthesiology www.abanes.org ; 919-881-2570?
   If a  nurse anesthetist is to administer the anesthetic, you can check  certification confirmation by contacting the American Association of Nurse Anesthetists at, www.aana.com; 847-692-7050, Ext. 1192. E-mail: certification@aana.com.

_____

_____

# The following questions apply to a CRNA or Physician Anesthesiologist and should be asked directly of the surgeon:

✔ How long have you worked with this specialist?

_____

_____

\*    For nearly all cosmetic procedures performed under general anesthesia, while you are asleep, the surgeon injects a local anesthetic into the operative site to induce tissue anesthesia and reduce bleeding.

✔  How long has the anesthesia specialist been practicing?
_____
_____

✔  Does the anesthesia specialist devote most or all of his time to cosmetic surgery cases?
_____
_____

✔  May I speak with the anesthesia specialist at any time prior to my procedure, to have specific concerns and questions answered?
_____
_____

✔  Will the anesthesia specialist conduct an independent review of my medical history?
_____
_____

✔  Who has the final say on whether or not the anesthesia can be conducted safely? The anesthesia specialist or my personal physician?
_____
_____

✔  How long after surgery will I awaken?
_____
_____

✔  How soon can I go home?
_____
_____

✔  Will the anesthesia specialist be present to assure my comfort and safety in the recovery room, following my procedure?
_____
_____

# Notes:

_____
_____
_____
_____
_____
_____
_____
_____
_____
_____
_____
_____
_____
_____
_____
_____
_____
_____
_____
_____
_____
_____
_____
_____
_____
_____
_____
_____
_____

Cosmetic Surgery Center records obtained by the state Department of Health list Ms. Lawrence as an anesthesia provider and say she administered Ketamine and Fentanyl. Investigators found no record that she had a nursing license in any state.

**— Dan O'Connor**
**"Woman Administered Anesthesia,**
**Assisted Surgeries Without Nursing License"**
_**Outpatient Surgery Magazine,**_
**September 2004**

Aesthetic surgeons must remain level-headed amid the frenzied atmosphere surrounding today's media coverage of cosmetic surgery. There is no excuse for allowing marketing hype to dictate practice standards. We must resist patient pressure for marathon surgeries beyond a reasonable number of hours. We must try to educate our patients about what is realistic for them — and for us as surgeons.

— **Stanley A. Klatsky, MD**
**Editor in Chief of** *Aesthetic Surgery Journal*
**"Surgical Marathons: Is Marketing Hype Dictating Practice Standards?"**
*Aesthetic Surgery Journal,* **May/June 2004**

I had an unnecessary and unfortunate experience. My doctor, who was an MD, FACS, told me that he would be administering my anesthesia. I did not know his assistant would be injecting into my face what felt like Novocain that did not last. So a series of injections were necessary. I had a restroom break halfway through the surgery. The surgery was a physically painful flop and an expensive experience financially, for which I had not planned. A year later I had a face surgery again by another doctor, also an MD, FACS, with a nurse anesthetist on staff. Days before surgery the nurse called me to review my medical history and assure me I would be comfortable during surgery. The surgery was successful and I look GREAT. It is a MUST to have an anesthesiologist or a nurse anesthetist with you on the day of surgery.

— **Gayle Y., Michigan**

## RIGHT BEFORE SURGERY — THE PRE-OP VISIT

After you've scheduled your procedure, there is a "countdown" period before the surgery day.

Most offices will schedule a face-to-face "pre-op visit" two to three weeks before surgery. This visit is important because it is an opportunity to have questions answered and to "nail down" all the scheduling and logistical details of the surgery day.

## Pre-operative Visit Checklist:

✔ Give your surgeon's office your night-before-surgery location and phone number or your cell phone so in case of a last-minute change in the surgery schedule, you can be contacted.

✔ Confirm that your history and physical, lab and X-ray tests have been performed, are normal and your primary care physician has given you the green light for elective surgery. Your surgeon's office should have received all reports.

✔ Confirm with the office that you will receive a call from the anesthesia specialist one or two nights prior to the surgery day. This is an opportunity for the anesthesiologist or anesthetist to discuss the anesthetic, answer your questions and best prepare you.

✔ Receive printed confirmation of the day, date, location and time of the surgery. If you have any uncertainty of the location of the surgical facility, ask for a map, directions and the surgical facility's phone number.

✔ You should receive printed instructions regarding:

  ✔ **Medications you *cannot* take** 7 to 10 days prior to surgery, e.g., aspirin.

  ✔ **Medications you *can* take** prior, e.g., routine maintenance medications such as thyroid, hormones, etc.

  ✔ **What food or drink can or cannot be consumed** in the 12-hour period prior to surgery.

  ✔ **Arrangements for postoperative care.** Who will be driving you home and caring for you and where? Be sure to clear this with the office.

✔ **Postoperative pain and other medications.** Will the office provide dressing supplies and pain medications? If not, you need to get prescriptions and a supply list so that you can have these in hand immediately after surgery.

✔ **Attention, smokers!** This is the perfect time to quit. Your surgeon will be happy; you will heal quicker. Your anesthesia specialist will be ecstatic; your anesthetic will go smoother; and you'll have a faster and less complicated recovery. If you can quit for the two-week period prior to surgery, can you not quit permanently?

# 8

# AFTER SURGERY —
## *Your Care Doesn't End with the Last Stitch*

After surgery, the critical period is always the first 24 hours. If major problems occur, most likely they or their harbingers will manifest within that time frame.

---

**Here are 15 questions to help put you at ease regarding the immediate post-operative period.**

### Post-Op Care Checklist

✔ What is the most common major problem that occurs in the immediate postoperative period?

_____

_____

✔ What about pain control?

_____

_____

✔ Given the procedure(s) I'm having, is it OK to recover at home, with a friend or relative in attendance, around the clock?

_____

_____

✔ Is a professional, e.g., RN, vocational nurse or nurse's aide, advisable?

_____

_____

✔ Do you offer a "recovery hideaway" facility as an alternative to recovering at home or at the home of a family member or friend?

_____

_____

✔ If so, what is the cost?

_____

_____

✔ How long a stay is recommended?

_____

_____

✔ May a family member or friend stay with me?

_____

_____

✔ May I visit the facility prior to my procedure?

_____

_____

✔ Does the facility provide transportation from the surgery center and to your office the next day?

_____

_____

✔ Will all the routine medications and supplies needed be provided, including pain medications, sleep medication and/or tranquilizers?

_____

_____

✔ I live 50 miles away. It takes more than one hour travel time; sometimes more during rush hour. Is it wise and safe for me to travel that distance after surgery?

_____

_____

✔ Speaking of distance, if I am that far away, and there is a problem, how will I be cared for? Shouldn't I stay closer to you and your office the first night? Perhaps a local hotel with friends and family?

_____

_____

✔ After surgery, at night, if I need to speak with you, how do I reach
you? Will I have your home phone number, your cell phone?

_____

_____

✔ If you are not available, who covers your practice and how do I
contact that doctor?

_____

_____

Satisfactory, comforting answers to the above 15 questions should put
you at ease. Remember, the doctor's care does not end with placement of
the last stitch. Top practices give attentive, personalized care before,
during and after the operating room.

## Notes:

# 9

# RATING THE PRACTICES
## *An Objective System for Making a Sound Evaluation*
### Cost Tabulation Worksheet

**Practice #1**

Doctor: _____
Phone: _____
E-Mail: _____
Fax: _____

Office Manager or Consultant:_____
Proposed Surgical Facility: _____

Recommended Procedure (s):                          Fees:
1. _____          $_____
2. _____          $_____
3. _____          $_____
4. _____          $_____
5. _____          $_____
6. _____          $_____
7. _____          $_____

                                    Subtotal:     $_____

Outpatient Surgery Center Charge                    $_____

Anesthesia Fee                                      $_____

Recovery Facility                                   $_____

Medications, Dressings                              $_____

                                    Total Cost:    $_____

# Cost Tabulation Worksheet

## Practice #2

Doctor: _____

Phone:_____

E-Mail:_____

Fax:_____

Office Manager or Consultant: _____

Proposed Surgical Facility:_____

Recommended Procedure (s):                          Fees:

1. _____    $_____
2. _____    $_____
3. _____    $_____
4. _____    $_____
5. _____    $_____
6. _____    $_____
7. _____    $_____

                               Subtotal:    $_____

Outpatient Surgery Center Charge             $_____

Anesthesia Fee                               $_____

Recovery Facility                            $_____

Medications, Dressings                       $_____

                             Total Cost:    $_____

# Cost Tabulation Worksheet

## Practice #3

Doctor: _____

Phone:_____

E-Mail:_____

Fax:_____

Office Manager or Consultant: _____

Proposed Surgical Facility:_____

Recommended Procedure (s):                         Fees:

1. _____     $_____

2. _____     $_____

3. _____     $_____

4. _____     $_____

5. _____     $_____

6. _____     $_____

7. _____   $_____

                              Subtotal:    $_____

Outpatient Surgery Center Charge              $_____

Anesthesia Fee                                        $_____

Recovery Facility                                     $_____

Medications, Dressings                              $_____

                         Total Cost:    $_____

## Take This Quiz to Score Any Cosmetic Surgery Practice

**Practice #1**        **Dr.** _____

### 1. The Initial Inquiry Via Telephone  (Maximum 6 Points)

**A.** Friendly, courteous, helpful?   (1 Point)        _____

**B.** Explains what the practice specializes in?  (1 Point)        _____

**C.** Offer to send more info?  (1 Point)        _____

**D.** Will give range of fees?   (1 Point)        _____

**E.** Lists the practice's six most frequently performed procedures?  (2 Points)        _____

### 2. The Educational Packet  (Maximum 4 Points)

**A.** Contains doctor's professional bio?  (1 Point)        _____

**B.** Map/directions to office?  (1 Point)        _____

**C.** Explains the office policy re consultation fee?  (1 Point)        _____

**D.** Describes the consultation process?  (1 Point)        _____

### 3. The Consultation  (Maximum 40 Points)

**A.** More time spent with doctor or staff member "consultant"?        _____
(4 Points if doctor; subtract 3 points if more time spent with consultant)

**B.** Computer imaging provided? (4 Points)        _____

**C.** Opportunity to see at least five "before-and-after" examples of the procedure(s) being considered?  (4 Points)        _____

**D.** Additional written info given to take home and study; i.e., frequently asked questions for the procedures, what to expect during the recovery period? (3 Points)        _____

**E.** Written quote given for all services, including surgeon's fee, anesthesia services and surgical facility? (2 Points)        _____

**F.** "Patient consultants" available? The office will pair you with one of its patients who is open and willing to discuss his experience? (4 Points) \_\_\_\_\_

**G.** A no-charge re-consultation is offered? (2 Points) \_\_\_\_\_

**H.** Gives you the choice of doctor-anesthesiologist or nurse-anesthetist? (4 Points) \_\_\_\_\_

**I.** Practice requires an independent, complete history and physical by your personal physician, internist or family physician? (4 Points) \_\_\_\_\_

**J.** Practice makes arrangements for you to speak with the anesthesia specialist prior to the day of surgery? (3 Points) \_\_\_\_\_

**K.** Practice will provide, as part of its service, at no additional cost to you, the routine medications and dressing supplies that you will require? (2 Points) \_\_\_\_\_

**L.** An explanation is given regarding charges if a secondary or touch-up surgery is necessary? (2 Points) \_\_\_\_\_

**M.** Will provide a list of medications (prescription and non-prescription) that could interfere with the anesthetic or surgical procedure? (2 Points) \_\_\_\_\_

## 4. The Doctor's Qualifications (Maximum 40 Points)

**A.** Board certified in one of the four specialties that are qualified to perform cosmetic surgery (dermatology, ophthalmology, head and neck surgery, plastic surgery)? (5 Points) \_\_\_\_\_

**B.** Practices cosmetic surgery only? (5 Points) \_\_\_\_\_

**C.** Completed a cosmetic surgery fellowship? (5 Points) \_\_\_\_\_

**D.** In his practice, performs only cosmetic surgery for 10 or more years? (5 Points) \_\_\_\_\_

**E.** Medical school faculty member, teaches cosmetic surgery? (5 Points) \_\_\_\_\_

**F.** Teaches other practicing doctors or cosmetic surgery trainees? (5 Points) \_\_\_\_\_

**G.** Has hospital privileges for both emergency admission and to perform his standard procedures? (5 Points) _____

**H.** Has written books and/or medical papers on cosmetic surgery? (5 Points) _____

## 5. The Office Staff (Maximum 10 Points)

**A.** Friendly, courteous and helpful? (2 Points) _____

**B.** Efficient? (2 Points) _____

**C.** Your appointment time was honored? (2 Points) _____

**D.** A staff member identified himself as the "contact person" for any further questions? (1 Point) _____

**E.** Pressure to schedule surgery? (If yes, **_deduct_** 10 Points) _____

**F.** Financial manager or consultant offered payment options including financing and credit card acceptance? (2 Points) _____

**G.** Discounts given for "friends and family" having procedures together; for "short notice" availability (standby); or if procedure is paid for far in advance? (1 Point) _____

TOTAL: _____

Maximum score =100

## Take This Quiz to Score Any Cosmetic Surgery Practice

**Practice #2**     **Dr.** _____

### 1. The Initial Inquiry Via Telephone  (Maximum 6 Points)

**A.** Friendly, courteous, helpful?   (1 Point)        _____

**B.** Explains what the practice specializes in?  (1 Point)        _____

**C.** Offer to send more info?  (1 Point)        _____

**D.** Will give range of fees?   (1 Point)        _____

**E.** Lists the practice's six most frequently performed
procedures?  (2 Points)        _____

### 2. The Educational Packet  (Maximum 4 Points)

**A.** Contains doctor's professional bio?  (1 Point)        _____

**B.** Map/directions to office?  (1 Point)        _____

**C.** Explains the office policy re consultation fee?  (1 Point)        _____

**D.** Describes the consultation process?  (1 Point)        _____

### 3. The Consultation  (Maximum 40 Points)

**A.** More time spent with doctor or staff member "consultant"?        _____
(4 Points if doctor; <u>subtract</u> 3 points if more time spent
with consultant)

**B.** Computer imaging provided? (4 Points)        _____

**C.** Opportunity to see at least five "before-and-after"
examples of the procedure(s) being considered?  (4 Points)        _____

**D.** Additional written info given to take home and
study; i.e., frequently asked questions for the procedures,
what to expect during the recovery period? (3 Points)        _____

**E.** Written quote given for all services, including surgeon's
fee, anesthesia services and surgical facility? (2 Points)        _____

**F.** "Patient consultants" available? The office will pair you with one of its patients who is open and willing to discuss his experience? (4 Points) _____

**G.** A no-charge re-consultation is offered? (2 Points) _____

**H.** Gives you the choice of doctor-anesthesiologist or nurse-anesthetist? (4 Points) _____

**I.** Practice requires an independent, complete history and physical by your personal physician, internist or family physician? (4 Points) _____

**J.** Practice makes arrangements for you to speak with the anesthesia specialist prior to the day of surgery? (3 Points) _____

**K.** Practice will provide, as part of its service, at no additional cost to you, the routine medications and dressing supplies that you will require? (2 Points) _____

**L.** An explanation is given regarding charges if a secondary or touch-up surgery is necessary? (2 Points) _____

**M.** Will provide a list of medications (prescription and non-prescription) that could interfere with the anesthetic or surgical procedure? (2 Points) _____

## 4. The Doctor's Qualifications (Maximum 40 Points)

**A.** Board certified in one of the four specialties that are qualified to perform cosmetic surgery (dermatology, ophthalmology, head and neck surgery, plastic surgery)? (5 Points) _____

**B.** Practices cosmetic surgery only? (5 Points) _____

**C.** Completed a cosmetic surgery fellowship? (5 Points) _____

**D.** In his practice, performs only cosmetic surgery for 10 or more years? (5 Points) _____

**E.** Medical school faculty member, teaches cosmetic surgery? (5 Points) _____

**F.** Teaches other practicing doctors or cosmetic surgery trainees? (5 Points) _____

**G.** Has hospital privileges for both emergency admission and to perform his standard procedures? (5 Points) _____

**H.** Has written books and/or medical papers on cosmetic surgery? (5 Points) _____

## 5. The Office Staff (Maximum 10 Points)

**A.** Friendly, courteous and helpful? (2 Points) _____

**B.** Efficient? (2 Points) _____

**C.** Your appointment time was honored? (2 Points) _____

**D.** A staff member identified himself as the "contact person" for any further questions? (1 Point) _____

**E.** Pressure to schedule surgery? (If yes, **_deduct_** 10 Points) _____

**F.** Financial manager or consultant offered payment options including financing and credit card acceptance? (2 Points) _____

**G.** Discounts given for "friends and family" having procedures together; for "short notice" availability (standby); or if procedure is paid for far in advance? (1 Point) _____

TOTAL: _____

**Maximum score = 100**

## Take This Quiz to Score Any Cosmetic Surgery Practice

**Practice #3**      **Dr. _____**

1. **The Initial Inquiry Via Telephone  (Maximum 6 Points)**

    **A.** Friendly, courteous, helpful?   (1 Point)          _____

    **B.** Explains what the practice specializes in?  (1 Point)          _____

    **C.** Offer to send more info?  (1 Point)          _____

    **D.** Will give range of fees?   (1 Point)          _____

    **E.** Lists the practice's six most frequently performed procedures?  (2 Points)          _____

2. **The Educational Packet  (Maximum 4 Points)**

    **A.** Contains doctor's professional bio?  (1 Point)          _____

    **B.** Map/directions to office?  (1 Point)          _____

    **C.** Explains the office policy re consultation fee?  (1 Point)          _____

    **D.** Describes the consultation process?  (1 Point)          _____

3. **The Consultation  (Maximum 40 Points)**

    **A.** More time spent with doctor or staff member "consultant"?          _____
    (4 Points if doctor; <u>subtract</u> 3 points if more time spent with consultant)

    **B.** Computer imaging provided? (4 Points)          _____

    **C.** Opportunity to see at least five "before-and-after" examples of the procedure(s) being considered?  (4 Points)          _____

    **D.** Additional written info given to take home and study; i.e., frequently asked questions for the procedures, what to expect during the recovery period? (3 Points)          _____

    **E.** Written quote given for all services, including surgeon's fee, anesthesia services and surgical facility? (2 Points)          _____

**F.** "Patient consultants" available?  The office will pair you with one of its patients who is open and willing to discuss his experience?  (4 Points)  _____

**G.** A no-charge re-consultation is offered?  (2 Points)  _____

**H.** Gives you the choice of doctor-anesthesiologist or nurse-anesthetist?  (4 Points)  _____

**I.** Practice requires an independent, complete history and physical by your personal physician, internist or family physician?  (4 Points)  _____

**J.** Practice makes arrangements for you to speak with the anesthesia specialist prior to the day of surgery?  (3 Points)  _____

**K.** Practice will provide, as part of its service, at no additional cost to you, the routine medications and dressing supplies that you will require?  (2 Points)  _____

**L.** An explanation is given regarding charges if a secondary or touch-up surgery is necessary?  (2 Points)  _____

**M.** Will provide a list of medications (prescription and non-prescription) that could interfere with the anesthetic or surgical procedure?  (2 Points)  _____

## 4. The Doctor's Qualifications  (Maximum 40 Points)

**A.** Board certified in one of the four specialties that are qualified to perform cosmetic surgery (dermatology, ophthalmology, head and neck surgery, plastic surgery)?  (5 Points)  _____

**B.** Practices cosmetic surgery only?  (5 Points)  _____

**C.** Completed a cosmetic surgery fellowship?  (5 Points)  _____

**D.** In his practice, performs only cosmetic surgery for 10 or more years?  (5 Points)  _____

**E.** Medical school faculty member, teaches cosmetic surgery?  (5 Points)  _____

**F.** Teaches other practicing doctors or cosmetic surgery trainees?  (5 Points)  _____

**G.** Has hospital privileges for both emergency admission and to perform his standard procedures? (5 Points) _____

**H.** Has written books and/or medical papers on cosmetic surgery? (5 Points) _____

## 5. The Office Staff  (Maximum 10 Points)

**A.** Friendly, courteous and helpful? (2 Points) _____

**B.** Efficient? (2 Points) _____

**C.** Your appointment time was honored? (2 Points) _____

**D.** A staff member identified himself as the "contact person" for any further questions? (1 Point) _____

**E.** Pressure to schedule surgery? ( If yes, **_deduct_** 10 Points) _____

**F.** Financial manager or consultant offered payment options including financing and credit card acceptance? (2 Points) _____

**G.** Discounts given for "friends and family" having procedures together; for "short notice" availability (standby); or if procedure is paid for far in advance? (1 Point) _____

TOTAL: _____

Maximum score = 100

Legally, any doctor can offer plastic surgery or cosmetic services regardless of his recognized board certification, training and skill level. This means that any medical doctor with the means or desire to market cosmetic surgery can do so without the proper training. Technically, your gynecologist or internist, or any licensed medical doctor, can perform a facelift, a breast lift or even inject Botox. Deciphering credentials can be confusing, and credentials alone are no guarantee. The difference among providers lies in their training and board certification by an appropriate medical specialty board recognized by the American Board of Medical Specialties (ABMS).  — **NewBeauty Magazine January 2005**

# 10

# HOMEWORK

## *After Your Consultations, You Still Need to Study and "Check Out a Few Things"*

## Information About Board Certification

**Q:** *What is the American Board of Medical Specialties?*

**A:** The **American Board of Medical Specialties** is the parent organization to the 24 official, approved medical specialty boards, including pediatrics, internal medicine, orthopedic surgery, obstetrics and gynecology. All 24 major specialties have a board to recognize its fully qualified practitioners. The **ABMS** coordinates the activities of its Member Boards and provides information to the public, the government, the profession and its members concerning issues involving specialization and certification of medical specialists.

Full board certification information is continually updated by the 24 Member Boards of the **ABMS**, including expiration information. Physicians review and update their own career and address information.

The latest edition includes information on nearly 600,000 board-certified physicians, in all 24 specialties; approximately 25,000 newly certified physicians are listed for the first time, and approximately 120,000 physicians have updated their listings.

For more information and the opportunity for you to confirm a physician's board certification in his specialty, contact:

**The American Board of Medical Specialties**
Phone: 847-491-9091
Phone Verification: 866-ASK-ABMS
Fax: 847-328-3596
www.abms.org

**Q:** *If a doctor is "board certified," what does that mean?*

**A:** Board certification is the medical profession's "stamp of approval." It verifies that the "diplomate" (holder of a board certification diploma) has met the standards of the profession to be qualified to present himself — to the profession and the public — as a fully qualified specialist.

The board-certified specialist has passed the test, literally and figuratively: oral and written examinations after successful completion of an approved residency in that particular specialty.

**Q:** *What does it mean if the doctor says he is "board qualified?"*

**A:** The "board qualified" doctor has completed an approved residency. Either he has not taken the exam or has failed the exam. Still eligible to take it again, the doctor is in a state of candidacy.

## The Four Boards Whose Diplomates May be Qualified to Perform Cosmetic Procedures Within Their Specialty

The following four boards are members of the **American Board of Medical Specialties** and are recognized as the official certifying boards for surgeons within those specialties.

**American Board of Dermatology**
The certifying board for dermatology
Phone: 313-874-1088
Fax: 313-874-3221
www.abderm.org

**American Board of Ophthalmology**
The certifying board for eye surgery
Phone: 610-664-1175
Fax: 610-664-6503
www.abop.org

**American Board of Otolaryngology**
The certifying board for otolaryngology-head and neck surgery
Phone: 713-850-0399
Fax: 713-850-1104
www.aboto.org

**American Board of Plastic Surgery**
The certifying board for plastic surgery
Phone: 215-587-9322
FAX: 215-587-9622
www.abplsurg.org

The following board is *not* a member of the **American Board of Medical Specialties.** It recognizes surgeons who practice surgery of the head and neck exclusively and who also have additional interest and knowledge of cosmetic and reconstructive surgery of the head and neck. This board administers certification examinations and has no involvement in the overseeing of residency training:

**American Board of Facial Plastic and Reconstructive Surgery**
Phone: 703-549-3223
Fax: 703-549-3357
www.abfprs.org

**Q:** *Is there no ABMS member board for cosmetic surgery only?*

**A:** There is not. Cosmetic surgery, a relatively new specialty, has no officially accepted board because there isn't a residency for cosmetic surgery only. No residency, no ABMS sanctioned board.

---

### Do your homework

In 1921 the need to screen out quacks and beauty "doctors" and certify reputable surgeons, even if they did perform cosmetic procedures, gave birth to the American Association of Plastic Surgeons. A decade later the American Society of Plastic and Reconstructive Surgeons (ASPRS) merged with it, and a few years after that the American Board of Plastic Surgery joined the association.

— **Ellen Feldman**
**"Before and After"**
*American Heritage,* **February/ March 2004**

---

> Consumers are already lost in a sea of data and tossed about like contradictory advice; they are like a rudderless ship in a storm.
> — **David H. McDaniel, MD**
> **Assistant Professor of Clinical**
> **Dermatology and Plastic Surgery,**
> **Eastern Virginia Medical School**
> *Cosmetic Surgery Times*, **October 2004**

# Specialty Organizations

These organizations provide additional educational material for prospective patients.

**American Academy of Dermatologic Surgery**
Phone: 847-956-0900
Fax: 847-956-0999
www.aboutskinsurgery.org

**American Academy of Dermatology**
Phone: 847-330-0230
Fax: 847-330-0050
www.aad.org

**The American Academy of Facial Plastic and Reconstructive Surgery**
Phone: 703-299-9291
Fax: 703-299-8898
www.aafprs.org

**The American Academy of Otolaryngology-Head and Neck Surgery**
Phone: 703-836-4444
Fax: 703-684-4288
www.entnet.org

**The American Society for Aesthetic Plastic Surgery**
Phone: 888) 272-7711
Fax: 562) 799-1098
www.surgery.org

**The American Society of Ophthalmic Plastic and Reconstructive Surgery**
Phone: 407-774-7880
Fax: 407-774-6440
www.asoprs.org

**The American Society of Plastic Surgeons**
Phone: 847-228-9900
Fax: 847-228-9131

www.plasticsurgery.org

# Surgery Facility Accreditation Organizations

The following are official accrediting organizations for surgical facilities in the United States. Facilities that hold one or more of these credentials are deemed "accredited."

**The Accreditation Association for Ambulatory Health Care (AAAHC)**
Phone: 847-853-6060
Fax: 847-853-9028
www.aaahc.org

**The American Association for Accreditation of Ambulatory Surgery Facilities (AAAASF)**
Phone: 847-775-1970
Fax: 847-775-1985
www.aaaasf.org

**The Joint Commission on Accreditation of Healthcare Organizations (JCAHO)**
Phone: 630-792-5000
Fax: 630-792-5005
www.jcaho.org

## United States Department of Health and Human Services (Medicare)

"Medicare Certification" signifies that the facility has met the U.S. government's standards to serve its Medicare patients. This credential is acceptable, with or without other credentials, for non-Medicare patients having cosmetic procedures.

## A State License to Operate a Medical Facility

If a facility holds a "state license" as an outpatient surgical facility, whether as a stand-alone building or within a medical or other building, it is considered to be duly accredited.

At consultation, ask if the facility in which the surgeon operates is "accredited." If not, beware! If it is, ask: "Accredited by whom?" The accreditation should be that of one of the above named organizations.

# Recommended Resources

## Magazines

*Allure*
www.allure.com

*Marie Claire*
www.marieclaire.com

*CosmoGIRL!*
www.hearst.com

*Men's Health*
www.menshealth.com

*Cosmopolitan*
www.cosmopolitan.com

*NewBeauty Magazine*
www.newbeauty.com

*Elle*
www.elle.com

*Self*
www.self.com

*Fitness*
www.fitnessmagazine.com

*Shape*
www.shape.com

*Glamour*
www.glamour.com

*Teen Vogue*
www.teenvogue.com

*In Style*
www.instyle.com

*Town and Country*
www.hearst.com

*Jane*
www.janemag.com

*Vogue*
www.vogue.com

*Marie Claire*
www.hearst.com

*W*
www.style.com/w

## Books

1. *THE LOWDOWN ON FACELIFTS & OTHER WRINKLE REMEDIES.* Wendy Lewis. Quadrille Publishing Ltd., London, England, 2001.

2. *THE BEAUTY BATTLE, An Insider's Guide to Wrinkle Rescue and Cosmetic Perfection from Head to Toe.* Wendy Lewis. Laurel Glen Publishing, San Diego, CA, 2002.

3. *THE MURAD METHOD, Wrinkle-Proof, Repair, and Renew Your Skin with the Proven 5-Week Program.* Murad Howard, MD. St. Martin's Press, New York, NY, 2003.

4. *100 QUESTIONS AND ANSWERS ABOUT PLASTIC SURGERY.* Diane Gerber, MD, FACS, and Marie Czenko Kuechel, MA. Jones and Bartlett Publishers, Sudbury, MA, 2005.

5. *LIFT. Wanting, Fearing, and Having a Face-Lift.* Joan Kron. Penguin Group, New York, NY, 1998.

6. *PLASTIC SURGERY HOPSCOTCH, A Resource Guide for Those Considering Cosmetic Surgery.* John McCabe. Edited by Miriam Ingersoll. Carmania Books, Santa Monica, CA, 1995.

7. *AGE-LESS, The Definitive Guide to Botox, Collagen, Lasers, Peels, and Other Solutions for Flawless Skin.* Fredric Brandt, MD, with Patricia Reynoso. Harper Collins Publishers, New York, NY, 2002.

8. *WHAT YOUR DOCTOR CAN'T TELL YOU ABOUT COSMETIC SURGERY.* Joyce D. Nash, PhD. toExcel, New York, NY, 2000.

9. *THE SMART WOMAN'S GUIDE TO PLASTIC SURGERY, Essential Information from a Female Plastic Surgeon.* Jean M. Loftus, MD. Contemporary Books, Chicago, Illinois, 2000.

10. *A LITTLE WORK, Behind the Doors of a Park Avenue Plastic Surgeon.* Z. Paul Lorenc, MD, FACS, and Trish Hall. St. Martin's Press, New York, NY, 2004.

11. *TWO GIRLFRIENDS GET REAL ABOUT COSMETIC SURGERY.* Charlee Ganny & Susan J. Collini. Renaissance Books, Los Angeles, CA, 2000.

12. *VENUS ENVY, A History of Cosmetic Surgery.* Elizabeth Haiken. Johns Hopkins University Press, Baltimore, Maryland, 1997.

13. *AMERICA'S COSMETIC DOCTORS AND DENTISTS: A Consumer Guide.* Wendy Lewis and John J. Connolly, Editors. Castle Connolly Medical, Ltd., New York, 2nd Edition, 2005

14. *COSMETIC SURGERY, THE CUTTING EDGE OF COMMERCIAL MEDICINE IN AMERICA.* Deborah Sullivan, Rutgers University Press, New Brunswick NJ, 2001.

15. *AESTHETIC SURGERY.* Angelika Taschen, Ed., Taschen, Cologne, 2005.

## Video Series

*The Naked Truth About Plastic Surgery,* a five-volume series edited by Garth Fisher, MD, FACS, the original *Extreme Makeover* plastic surgeon. The section on chemical skin peels was contributed by yours truly. Available at www.nakedtruth.com.

## Web Sites

www.iVillage.com  www.robertkotlermd.com
www.beautysurg.com  www.surgerysecrets.com
www.webMD.com  www.cosmeticsurgery-news.com

## JUST TO BE SURE ...
## You can verify the doctor is licensed and in good standing.

Once in a while, you read about or watch an exposé of a "bogus doctor." Yes, there are clever scam artists and con men out there preying on patients. These quacks typically practice in neighborhood or storefront clinics or even have no office, performing minor procedures, usually the less invasive ones such as filling injections or Botox, in their residence or at a patient's residence. The scrutiny of the medical profession's credentialing processes bars them from licensed hospitals and accredited outpatient surgery centers.

If you follow this book's advice, it's not likely a fake doctor will pass your scrutiny. But if anything you see, hear or just have a gut feeling about gives you discomfort, do one single thing: Check with the medical board of your state or in the state in which the doctor would care for you. Confirm that "Dr. X" is indeed a licensed physician. To locate the appropriate state medical board, contact:

Federation of State Medical Boards of the United States Inc.
P.O. Box 619850
Dallas, TX 75261-9850
phone 817-868-4000; fax 817-868-4098; http://www.fsmb.org

If the board confirms that the doctor is licensed and thus not a fraud, you can also ask if Dr. X's license is "current and unrestricted." Confirm that there is no current disciplinary activity in place against him. One short call. You'll sleep better.

---

The Federation of State Medical Boards of the United States, Inc., is a national organization composed of the 70 medical boards of the United States, the District of Columbia, Puerto Rico, Guam and the U.S. Virgin Islands. On behalf of its membership, FSMB's mission is to improve the quality, safety and integrity of health care through the development and promotion of high standards for physician licensure and practice.

---

# APPENDIX A

## Glossary: The Language of Cosmetic Surgery

The world of cosmetic enhancement has its own language; a unique lingo. To best communicate with the doctor and his staff, here is a list of the most commonly used terms, courtesy Wendy Lewis, author of *THE LOWDOWN ON FACELIFTS & OTHER WRINKLE REMEDIES*, an excellent resource.

**Ablation:** Vaporization of the most superficial layers of skin.

**Acne:** Chronic condition characterized by an inflammatory eruption of the skin.

**Arnica:** A botanical derived from a mountain plant with antiseptic, astringent, antimicrobial and anti-inflammatory properties.

**Asymmetry:** Differences in the two sides of the face or in individual parts of the face that are in pairs, e.g. the eyes, the brows, etc.

**Bleaching agents:** Slowing down or blocking the production of melanin to lighten age spots and fade areas of hyperpigmentation, e.g. kojic acid, hydroquinone.

**Blepharoplasty:** Surgery to rejuvenate the upper and/or lower eyelids by removing fatty or excess tissue from the eyelids.

**Botox® Cosmetic:** The brand name for botulinium toxin, that is injected into the muscles to smooth out wrinkles by temporarily paralyzing the muscles that cause contraction.

**Brow lift:** A surgical procedure in which drooping eyebrows are elevated to a higher position.

**Cannula:** Long, thin hollow tubular instrument used to extract fat during liposuction.

**Carbon dioxide laser:** Laser technology used to resurface facial wrinkles and scars. Also can be used as a cutting tool in surgery.

**Cheek augmentation:** A procedure designed to give more definition to the cheekbones by implanting artificial materials or grafting bone into the malar region.

**Cheek lift:** Also referred to as the "mid-facelift," this is a surgical procedure designed to lift sagging areas in the mid-face, including around the cheek-bone area below the eyes.

**Chemical peeling:** Skin resurfacing, when a chemical solution is applied to the skin so that the top skin layer will peel off.

**Chin augmentation:** A surgical procedure to build up a recessive chin by inserting a solid silicone rubber implant material or by grafting bone to the chin.

**Collagen:** Component of human skin that gives it resilience, suppleness and tone. It breaks down with age.

**Collagen instant therapy:** Injectable purified collagen extracted from cowhide.

**Composite lift:** An operation designed to lift the skin and underlying soft tissue of the face, brow and upper eyelids; also referred to as the deep-plane facelift.

**Corrugator:** Muscle that is responsible for causing the glabellar or vertical lines that form between the eyebrows.

**Cosmeceutical:** A substance that falls between the classification of a drug and a cosmetic, i.e. non-prescription over-the-counter formulations that provide pharmaceutical benefits.

**Crow's-feet:** Wrinkles around the outer corners of the eyes.

**Dermabrasion:** A form of skin resurfacing that aims to improve irregular or uneven skin texture and acne scars.

**Dermis:** The layer of skin composed of collagen and elastin, lying beneath the epidermis (outer layer) and above the subcutaneous layers of skin.

**Dissect:** To separate anatomical structures via controlled tearing or cutting through the connective tissue that holds them together.

**Drainage:** A tube that is inserted in or near a surgical wound to drain excess blood and fluid.

**Dry eye:** A condition of the eyelids caused by low tear production and manifested by dryness, inflammation, irritation and blurred vision of the eyes.

**Ectropion:** A condition of the lower eyelid in which the lid is pulled downward by loose eyelid skin or muscles or from having too much skin removed; also called "lid retraction."

**Edema:** Swelling or fluid retention that can occur after surgery or inflammation.

**Embolus:** A piece of blood clot, fat or air bubble that breaks away and can infiltrate the bloodstream during surgery.

**Endoscopically assisted surgery:** A small, rigid, tube-like instrument called an endoscope is equipped with fiberoptic lighting and can be introduced into the body through a tiny incision to light up the surgical area shown on a video monitor while the surgeon performs the operation, as in endoscopic browlifting, facelifting, etc.

**Epithelialization:** Regeneration of the epithelium or superficial layer of the skin, as occurs after laser resurfacing.

**Erythema:** Redness of the skin caused by increased blood flow to the area, as in post-laser or other resurfacing treatments.

**Excision:** Removal via surgical cutting.

**Exfoliant:** A material that removes dead surface skin cells.

**Extrusion:** The erosion of skin that causes an implant (chin, lip, breast, etc.) to become partially exposed.

**Facelift:** A surgical operation designed to reposition and support sagging skin and its underlying tissues, and to remove excess skin and fat. Term usually indicates the lifting of the lower two-thirds of the face and neck, but does not include the eyes or the forehead.

**Fascia:** The sheet of connective tissue that covers the muscles, sometimes used as a graft material.

**Frontalis:** Main forehead muscle that elevates brows and contributes to the formation of horizontal wrinkles of the forehead.

**Glabellar:** The region between the eyebrows.

**Graft:** A piece of tissue that is removed from one part of the body and transferred to another area of the body.

**Hematoma:** A localized accumulation of blood in the skin caused by a blood vessel wall rupture; a possible complication of surgery that may have to be drained out.

**Hyperpigmentation:** An excess of pigment in a skin area causes darkness; also can be caused by sun exposure.

**Hypopigmentation:** Reduction in the pigment cells in the skin resulting in skin lightening; can occur after resurfacing.

**Keloid:** The overgrowth of fibrous scar tissue

**Laser:** Acronym for Light Amplification by the Simulated Emission of Radiation, a device that emits an intense beam that can be precisely directed and controlled.

**Laser skin resurfacing:** Treatment of skin conditions with a laser, so that a beam of light is focused to penetrate or vaporize tissues. Laser skin resurfacing is used to improve wrinkles, to treat facial veins and to remove sunspots, facial hair, port-wine stains and certain kinds of tattoos.

**Lateral hooding:** Excess fold of skin between the eyebrow and the outer portion of the upper eyelid.

**Liposuction:** The removal of fat with a slender hollow instrument called a cannula. This instrument is inserted through a very small incision and attached to a suction machine to vacuum out excessive fat.

**Lymphatic system:** A network of structures, including ducts and nodes, that carry lymph fluid from tissues to the bloodstream.

**Malar bags:** The pouch of loose skin and fluid that sometimes occurs with age below the lower eyelid area.

**Malar fat pad:** A structure that sits in the second layer of the face below the cheekbone that is frequently repositioned during facial rejuvenation procedures.

**Marionette lines:** The vertical creases that form in the corners of the mouth and jowls.

**Mentoplasty:** A shaping or molding of the chin, such as building up the chin through chin augmentation.

**Micro-dermabrasion:** Mechanical blasting of the face with sterile micro particles that abrade or rub off the top layer of skin, after which the particles and dead cells are vacuumed away.

**Monitoring devices:** Operating room equipment that is used to closely watch and report the body's vital functions, e.g. heart rate, pulse, oxygen, blood pressure.

**Nasal labial fold:** The crease or fold of skin and soft tissues that runs from the outer corners of the upper lip.

**Necklift:** A surgical operation to lift sagging tissues of the neck and tighten the underlying musculature.

**Orbicularis oculi:** The muscular body of the eyelid encircling the eye and compromising the palpebral, orbital and lacrimal muscles. The orbital muscle functions to close the eyelids which causes wrinkling or crow's-feet.

**Phenol:** Acid-like chemical applied to the skin to lighten pigment, soften wrinkles and improve scars, considered to be a deep and more invasive peel.

**Photoaging:** Skin damage caused by cumulative exposure to the sun's rays, i.e. wrinkles, age spots, fine lines, etc.

**Platysmal band:** Vertical strands of the muscle of the neck that can become more prominent with age and are often sutured or tightened during a facelift.

**Plication:** A surgical technique that involves tucking or pleating.

**Procerus:** Muscle that works with the corrugator muscles and contributes to the vertical frown lines between the eyebrows.

**Ptosis:** Pronounced "toe-sis," a term for drooping as in eyelids, breasts and brows.

**Rhytidectomy:** Technical term for a facelift.

**Saline:** Salt water commonly used as a filler for breast implants and in the course of administering intravenous fluids.

**Scleral show:** Lower eyelid retraction that exposes the sclera (white part of the eyeball) below the pupil.

**Seroma:** A collection of clear fluid that may develop following surgery.

**Silastic sheeting:** Patches or strips of silicone that may be applied to the skin for extended periods to soften and reduce scarring.

**Silicone:** A synthetic substance used in a gel-like form in breast implants; in a liquid-injectable form for facial areas; and in other medical devices.

**SMAS:** Acronym for the Superficial Musculo-Aponeurotic System; a layer of tissue that covers the deeper structures in the cheek area and touches the superficial muscle covering the lower face and neck, called the platysma.

**Steroids:** Any of a large number of hormonal substances with similar basic chemical structure, produced mainly in the adrenal cortex and gonads.

**Subcutaneous:** Under the skin.

**Submental:** The area below the chin.

**Subperiosteal:** A term for a facelift procedure that goes deep into multiple layers; a lift in which all tissues are separated from the underlying bone structure, thereby considered more invasive.

**Tragus:** A small extension of the auricular cartilage of the ear, anterior to the external meatus.

**Tumescent:** A method of anesthesia in which large volumes of local anesthetic and saline solution are injected to swell the area to be operated on; commonly used in liposuction and body-contouring procedures.

**Undermining:** Surgical separation of tissues from their underlying structures.

# APPENDIX B

# THE 29 MOST IMPORTANT
# COSMETIC SURGERY CONSULTATION
# QUESTIONS

| QUESTION | YES | NO | NOTES |
|---|---|---|---|
| 1. Is the majority of the doctor's practice devoted to cosmetic surgery? | | | |
| 2. What percentage of the doctor's practice is cosmetic vs. reconstructive plastic surgery? | | | |
| 3. How long has the doctor been performing the procedure you are considering? | | | |
| 4. How many of these procedures has he performed? | | | |
| 5. Did the doctor learn to perform this procedure as part of his formal residency training, or did he learn it after he completed his residency when he was in practice? | | | |
| 6. Is the doctor board certified? Which board or boards? | | | |
| 7. Has the doctor completed a full-time, six-month-to-one-year cosmetic surgery fellowship? | | | |
| 8. Is the doctor a Fellow of the American College of Surgeons? | | | |
| 9. Is the doctor or has the doctor been a medical school faculty member? | | | |
| 10. Is the doctor a member of local, state and national medical societies? Which ones? | | | |
| 11. Has the doctor written books or authored journal articles on the cosmetic surgery procedure(s) you are considering? | | | |
| 12. Does the doctor teach other doctors his techniques of cosmetic surgery? | | | |
| 13. How many of these procedures does the doctor perform in an average week? | | | |

| QUESTION | YES | NO | NOTES |
|---|---|---|---|
| **14.** Does the doctor have hospital privileges to perform the procedure you are considering? | | | |
| **15.** Does the doctor have hospital admitting privileges in case of emergency? | | | |
| **16.** Is the surgery performed entirely by your surgeon? Or is part delegated to a surgeon-in-training? | | | |
| **17.** Will the doctor and the staff perform all postoperative care? | | | |
| **18.** Can you receive a copy of the doctor's professional biography that summarizes his training, qualifications and credentials? | | | |
| **19.** Where will the procedure be done? If in the doctor's office, has the operating room and recovery room been accredited by a recognized authority, e.g., the Joint Commission on Accreditation of Health Care Organizations (JCAHO), the Accreditation Association for Ambulatory Health Care (AAAHC), or the American Association for Accreditation of Ambulatory Surgical Facilities (AAAASF)? | | | |
| **20.** If in an outpatient or ambulatory surgery center, is the center licensed by the state and/or certified by the U.S. government? By JCAHO, AAAHC or AAAASF? | | | |
| **21.** Is the outpatient surgical facility located in a medical building? | | | |
| **22.** Will the anesthetic be administered by an anesthesiologist (physician specialist), nurse anesthetist or the surgeon? | | | |
| **23.** Is a recovery "hideaway" and transportation to and from the office available? | | | |
| **24.** Are typical "before-and-after" photos made available for your viewing? Do the results look natural? Is the improvement significant? | | | |
| **25.** Does the office provide "computer imaging" to help you visualize the anticipated results of your procedure(s)? | | | |

| QUESTION | YES | NO | NOTES |
|---|---|---|---|
| **26.** Can you speak and/or meet with a patient who has had surgery performed by the doctor? | | | |
| **27.** Does the office provide, at the consultation, an itemized "fee quotation sheet" listing all proposed services and charges? | | | |
| **28.** Does the office offer a financing program? | | | |
| **29.** What is the policy regarding charges for touch-up surgery? | | | |

*We don't know what we don't know. To know, we must know the right questions to ask.*
— **A. Norman Enright**
**E-5 U.S. Coast Guard, 1965**

*There are no dumb questions. Except the the ones my husband asks.*
— **Louise Epstein**
**Green Lake, WI**

**When to Walk**
### Nine Sure Signs That a Doctor Is Not the One for You

1. If the doctor is willing to perform surgery without an initial health evaluation.

2. If you are not given, prior to treatment, pre- and post-procedure instructions and cautions.

3. If your doctor trivializes the risks involved with your procedure.

4. If the doctor makes unrealistic guarantees or promises.

5. If the doctor is willing to perform or suggests unrelated, multiple, extensive procedures. Remember, an Extreme Makeover marathon of surgery, like a tummy tuck, liposuction, breast procedure and facelift, in one surgical session puts you at risk.

6. If the doctor tells you what you need before listening to what you want.

7. If the office, doctor or staff are disorganized and disheveled.

8. If pricing is not outlined prior to treatment. The only variables in pricing should be related to operating room time, anesthesia and unexpected events.

9. If anyone other than the doctor who will perform your procedure examines you and defines a course of treatment.

— *NewBeauty Magazine,* January 2005

# APPENDIX C

## COMPANIES THAT FINANCE COSMETIC SURGERY:

**Advanced Patient Financing**
Toll-Free: 877-275-7526
www.apsportfolio.com

**AmeriCharge**
American General Finance
8929 Sepulveda Blvd., #100
Los Angeles, CA 90045
800-599-8653
Fax: 310-641-8653
www.agfinance.com

**CareCredit**
901 E. Cerritos Ave.
Anaheim, CA 92805
800-839-9078
Fax: 714-491-7005
www.carecredit.com

**Cosmetic Fee Plan**
Toll-Free: 888-440-2379
www.cosmeticfeeplan.com

**Cosmetic Surgery Financing**
Toll-Free: 888-405-8140
www.cosmeticsurgeryfinanc
ing.com/ba

**Health Capital Finance Group**
1077 Bridgeport Ave.
Shelton, CT 06484
800-637-8324
Fax: 800-466-0043
www.patientfinance.com

**Health Ready**
Toll-Free:
888-873-1082
www.healthready.com

**MediCredit**
5150 E. Pacific Coast Hwy., #570
Long Beach, CA 90804
800-963-6334
Fax: 800-987-3299
www.medicredit.com

**Monarch Patient Finance**
Toll-Free: 888-230-1600
www.monarchfinance.com

**PFS Patient Finance**
908-754-2500
Toll-Free: 888-737-3679
Fax:908-754-9192
www.p-f-s.com

**Reliance Finance Corporation**
9911 W. Pico Blvd., Suite 1200
Los Angeles, CA 90035
310-551-0988
800-322-6377
Fax: 310-551-0989
www.reliancemedicalfinance.com

**SurgeryLoans.com**
16 Technology Dr.
Suite 173
Irvine, CA 92618
888-502-8020
Fax: 888-502-8030
www.surgeryloans.com

**Unicorn Patient Financing**
Toll-Free: 888-388-7633
www.unicornfinancial.com

**Hint:** Ask the office manager which company or companies have given their patients the best service. You will be signing a loan document: Read the fine print, and it's not a bad idea to run it by a financial professional or an attorney.

# APPENDIX D

# THE POPULAR ACCESSORIES:
## Botox® Cosmetic and the Fillers and Plumpers

### The Fillers and Plumpers

Science is delivering a host of good products to improve facial structure, soften the effects of aging, and help restore youthful appearance. With the introduction of collagen injections in the late 1970s, an armory of efficient products began to be built. These injectable, so-called "fillers" or "plumpers" are commonly used to plump thin lips, fill the naso-labial groove (oblique trough between the cheek, laterally, and the nose and lip, medially). They also are used to correct the "puppet line" groove that extends vertically from the outer corners of the lower lip, separating the cheek, laterally, from the chin, medially.

For younger female patients, the lip plumping role is more popular. For the middle aged and "older" men and women, filling the naso-labial groove is the main mission. For male patients, whose core knowledge of cosmetic procedures lags behind that of females, when I explain the need to fill the naso-labial groove or puppet line, I call upon the proper noun, "Bondo." Immediately comes forth the affirmative up-and-down head nod; a man gets it. He understands the concept. Bondo, for all you female readers, is the universally known filling compound that auto body shops employ to fill dents and dings. Both Bondo and filling injections plump dents and dings. A technical distinction is that Bondo is applied to the auto body surface. Cosmetic injections "lift" the skin's surface when the filler is injected below it. Hence the plumping effect.

### Why So Many Filling Materials?

There is an axiom that lives in every doctor's brain. It is learned early in his education. "When there are many solutions to a given condition, no single solution is ideal." Each has strengths, and weaknesses, which is why there is a wide variety of fillers for a variety of indications.

The ideal filling material, were it to exist, would exhibit these qualities:

- Painless introduction.
- Even distribution within the tissue.

- Little reactivity; e.g., no redness, swelling, discomfort or bruising.
- Permanence.
- Inexpensive.

That is the wish list, of course.

If you ask patients what single quality they value most in such procedures, I suspect it is permanence. But permanence is good and bad. Here is why.

## The Case for Absorbable, Nonpermanent Fillers

I advise patients to consider the great virtue of the absorbable, nonpermanent filler injection. You get to rent it but not own it. You demo it. You decide if you like the look or not and, most importantly, how much of it is ideal for your appearance and for your wallet.

Patients can get comfortable with their appearance without worrying about it being "overdone." The ideal method is to ask the doctor or nurse to inject a reasonable amount and see how it looks after a week or so, when whatever injection-induced swelling there is disappears. If you want more, you stop into the doctor's office for a "topping off." And, if the initial injection was a bit generous for your liking, well, relax. It is not permanent, it will dissipate within several months, and next time you will "order less."

Yes, permanence is convenient, but once injected, a permanent material cannot be withdrawn. "It's done."

But remember the flip side: "What if?" If too much of a permanent solution is injected into your lips, for example, and you are now sporting trout lips, you are stuck with them. Not cool unless you're a fish.

## Remember Kotler's Caveat:

Whenever possible, "try before you buy." Vote for a "demo" whenever you can; try absorbable products like collagen or hyaluronic acid, because permanent fillers, like liquid silicone, cannot be extracted or removed. Why paint yourself into a corner?

# My Short List of the Most Popular and Important Fillers and Plumpers

**Collagen Injections**—Collagen is a naturally occurring substance in the skin and a principle contributor to the skin's strength and smoothness. It can be used to improve facial lines, creases, grooves and some scars. Collagen injections are used as "fillers." They also work for "indentations," such as the deep crease between the cheeks and lip. The substance is injected into and underneath the skin and takes effect immediately. Because it is derived from animal tissue that is not living, the body digests and eliminates it. Therefore, it is necessary for your doctor to perform "refills" every three or four months. Collagen has been available for more than 20 years and has proven itself to be safe, practical and effective. Zyplast® and Zyderm®, from Inamed Aesthetics, require skin testing to disprove allergy. Cosmoplast® and Cosmoderm®, Inamed's newer products, do not require skin testing.

**Fat Injections**—Fat injection techniques are still in a state of evolution. Theoretically, fat would be an ideal substance to fill deep creases and grooves in the face, thereby replacing the missing fat, which shrinks in the natural course of aging. However, the perfect solution for using fat transplantation has proven to be somewhat elusive. Using a liposuction-type technique the fat is harvested from hidden areas, such as the lower abdomen or buttocks. It is then injected into the facial areas that need it. The challenge of this procedure has been to perfect the technique so as to maximize transplanted fat survival, minimize absorption and eliminate lumpiness and irregularities.

**Hyaluronic Acid**—Hyaluronan is a naturally occurring substance in our bodies. As we get older, hyaluronan decreases and the skin becomes less taut and more dry. When injected into the skin, Hyaluronic acid increases the level of hyaluronan. Since there is no species specificity, no skin testing is necessary. Restylane® and Hylaform® gel are the two most frequently used, approved, hyaluronic acid products. Perlane®, a similar but thicker substance, awaits FDA approval.

**Silicone**—Medical-grade silicone is a clear, oil-like liquid that has been successfully used to fill grooves, depressions and raised scars on the face for decades. Because of the silicone breast implant controversy, many practitioners abandoned it. However, silicone in experienced hands can be safe and effective. Recently, Silicone 1000 (Alcon Corporation) was approved for certain medical uses. Cosmetic surgeons use it for many indications, including the treatment of certain types of wrinkles and acne scars. Because silicone is permanent and cannot be removed, be sure that your desires are reasonable, practical and wise.

## Botox® Cosmetic and Myobloc™

Treatment of hyperfunctional lines with botulinum toxin occupies a unique and welcome role in facial rejuvenation. Neither Botox® Cosmetic nor Myobloc™ "fills in" nor "puffs out" grooves and creases; they are not filling materials. These muscle weakeners are very effective on the forehead and between the eyebrows, the site of strong, repeated muscle contraction. The drug's paralyzing effect temporarily blocks nerve transmission, thereby lessening muscle tension and relaxing the tissues.

Botox® Cosmetic and Myobloc™ are office treatments. The result takes three to five days to manifest, and the benefits last from three to six months. Some surgeons are experimenting with Botox® Cosmetic to reduce prominence of the vertical muscle cords of the neck (platysma bands).

---

### Questions You Must Ask Your Doctor
### Before Any Treatment with Injectables

1. Are you a board-certified plastic surgeon, facial plastic surgeon or dermatologist?

2. Exactly what name brand and amount of injectable will you be using, and where will you inject it?

3. How long have you been using this type of injectable, and will you personally provide the treatment?

4. How many people have you treated with a similar condition, and may I see photographs of before-and-after results?

5. What type or combination of injection therapies do you recommend to address my concerns?

---

# TEN QUESTIONS TO ASK IF YOU ARE THINKING ABOUT RECEIVING BOTOX COSMETIC THERAPY *

by Wm. Philip Werschler, MD
Clinical Professor, University of Washington

You believe that appearance is a priority in your life, and are concerned about looking your best. You either don't want or don't feel that invasive surgery (e.g., facelift) is necessary. For now, you would like to focus on minimal downtime procedures, and for those worrisome frown lines between your eyebrows, those annoying crow's-feet, and that furrowed brow, Botox is the best thing going.

Once you make the decision to get Botox therapy, how do you go about doing it properly? First, make sure that you understand just what Botox therapy can and can't do for you. Botox is not a filling substance like collagen, and it does not directly affect the skin. Botox is a natural purified protein that, when gently placed into the skin with a tiny needle, relaxes and smooths the targeted muscle(s). Over time, this will result in a softening of dynamic skin folds (deep wrinkles) and lessen your ability to move the muscles involved in making these lines. This can and will affect your ability to make certain expressions, particularly frowning.

**The Top 10 list of questions for successful Botox therapy:**

Ask yourself:

- **Am I pregnant or breast-feeding?** If so, sorry, no Botox. You already look heavenly, so wait until you and Mother Nature have completed your mission before getting this therapy.

- **Do I have any neuromuscular disease?** If the answer is yes, or you are not sure, check with your treating physician or a neurologist to see if Botox therapy is safe for you.

* *Healthy Skin and Hair*, Summer 2002

✔ **Am I taking any aminoglycoside antibiotics or neuromuscular medications?** If you think so, or don't know, find out before receiving Botox therapy.

✔ **Do I have any active skin disease (acne cysts, infections, rashes, etc.) at the site of the injection?** Because Botox is administered with a needle, if you have any of these, you probably need to see a dermatologist for treatment prior to getting Botox therapy.

✔ **Am I prepared to change my facial appearance, albeit temporarily?** If you're not sure about this one, you need to think it over, or better yet, talk to someone who already has had Botox therapy. Trust me, they won't be hard to find.

Ask your physician:

✔ **How much experience do you have with Botox therapy for facial lines?** While Botox treatments are not brain surgery, they are not for amateur injectors, either. Whoever delivers your treatments should be, at minimum, trained in facial anatomy, with a comprehensive understanding of the muscles of facial expression and their response to Botox. Typically, these are the offices of dermatologists, facial plastic surgeons, and oral-maxillofacial surgeons.

✔ **How do you charge for Botox?** Treatments always should be charged by the volume, in units, of Botox used. This way, everyone pays for the amount they actually use. Some offices also may charge an additional injection fee or office visit charge. If the office charges everybody the same fee for the same areas treated, such as the forehead, then people with big foreheads are getting a good deal, and those with small foreheads are probably being overcharged. Insist on paying only for what you use.

✔ **How are touch-up treatments handled?** No matter how much experience an injector has, not every patient reacts the same, and on occasion, "touch-ups" are necessary to even out results or to achieve the best possible improvement. Some offices charge for this, and others don't, so be sure to ask.

✔ **Is the dilution of Botox used kept constant?** Many different dilutions are used in the United States, and they typically range from 1.0 cc to 10 cc. If you are being charged by the unit of Botox, as you should, then the dilution used should not matter in terms of price and performance. In this case, 20 units in a 2 cc dilution is the same as 20 units in a 3 cc dilution. Beware of the "Botox sale," as the number of units injected may be less to reflect the lowered price. Remember, you never get something for nothing.

✔ **Finally, remember the old saying "caveat emptor" or "buyer beware."** With the recent FDA approval of Botox Cosmetic, there will no doubt be a rush of new "Botox Injectors" springing up . If the Botox ad sounds too good to be true, it probably is. Allergan, the manufacturer of Botox Cosmetic, has a Web site (www.BotoxCosmetic.net) and a toll-free phone number (800-BotoxMD) for the Botox Cosmetic Physicians' Network. Stick with these experienced and reputable medical practices, and you should experience a great result with your Botox therapy.

# A SPECIAL OFFER

## Did We Forget An Important Question?

If we did, and you think it is important enough for others to know about it, send us the question and we'll return the favor by sending you a personally autographed copy of Dr. Kotler's best-seller, *SECRETS OF A BEVERLY HILLS COSMETIC SURGEON, The Expert's Guide to Safe Successful Surgery.*

Our way of saying "thanks" for helping us educate the public.

**~Ernest Mitchell Publishers**

If you would like to order
*The Essential Cosmetic Surgery Companion*
as a gift to a friend, loved one or colleague,
please go to our website
www.robertkotlermd.com
or to your favorite bookseller.

# The only other book you must have if you're seriously considering cosmetic surgery.

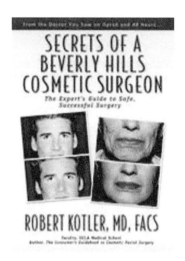

Dr. Robert Kotler, not only guides you through the entire decision process—he also dispels many common myths and misconceptions about face and body surgery. Dr. Kotler reveals:

- Why some celebrities look so bad after cosmetic surgery.

- That most surgical fees are negotiable—and while sky-high fees do not guarantee superior results, low-ball fees may not be a bargain.

- Why some self-proclaimed "cosmetic surgeons" are poorly trained, unqualified and may be practicing on you.

- How some medications, vitamins and herbs can speed healing while others, including the 136 you do not want to take, are dangerous.

*"For anyone who is considering enhancing their physical appearance via cosmetic surgery, this book will tell you everything you need to know. The information will give you more confidence in making the right choices – from how to select your doctor to what procedure is best suited for your specific needs…what to expect during a specific procedure, especially the recovery process, as well as what mental blocks you may possibly experience."*

**~ Lillian Glass, PhD,**
**Best selling author, counseling psychologist, and**
**communication expert**

# Read What Authorities are Saying About
*SECRETS OF A BEVERLY HILLS COSMETIC SURGEON*
*The Expert's Guid*e to Safe, Successful Surgery

*"If you're thinking of cosmetic surgery or just want to learn more, this is the book. Dr. Kotler, one of the top cosmetic surgeons in the United States, guides you through the procedures and what each entails-from costs to recovery times. You will truly be informed..."*
**~ Mary Ann Malloy, MD Women's health expert, NBC**

*"Cosmetic surgery can be a life-changing decision, and Dr. Kotler relays valuable information so the public can make an informed decision. An excellent resource for both doctor and patient. Sound decisions translate to peace of mind an important, factor when considering plastic surgery."*
**~ Howard Murad, MD**
**Assistant Clinical Professor of Dermatology, UCLA**

*"The secrets of finding a cosmetic surgeon who is right, for you. A must have book for anyone contemplating this type of surgery."*
**~ Dr. Earl Mindell**
**Author, Vitamin, Herb and Diet Bibles**

*''Dr. Robert Kotler, an acknowledged master of facial plastic surgery has written an informative, easy, 1vell-organized and humorous `must read' for the patient who requires education regarding cosmetic surgery in order to be well versed in all nuances and protected from the pitfalls."*
**~ Jeremy L. Freeman, MD**
**Professor of Otolaryngology, University of Toronto**

*"A bible for the consumer who is looking for rejuvenation, and is concerned about what procedure they really need and who's the best to do it. Contains checklists to make sure they stay on the right track."*
**~ James E. Fulton Jr., MD, PhD, Co-Developer Retin-A®**

*"A thorough consumer's guide highlighting all important areas one should consider when contemplating cosmetic surgery. Consumers should do their homework, and this book is invaluable toward that end."*
**~ David B. Barinholtz, MD,**
**Clinical Associate University of Chicago,**
**Pritzker School of Medicine**

*"Complete and concise. In today's complex cosmetic surgery world, there are more choices for procedures, operating facilities and surgeons. That's why the consumer needs this book."*
**~ Kurt J. Wagner, MD, FACS**
**Board Certified Plastic Surgeon**

## SAMPLE THIS SPECIAL BOOK
## RIGHT NOW

This 258 page, hardcover book, includes over 50 case histories, illustrated with dramatic before and after photos.

**Chapter 1,** an overview of the entire book, is reprinted for your convenience. In **Chapter 1, Snapshot of the Big Picture**, you'll find Dr. Kotler's clear and insightful explanation of why some celebrities look so bad after cosmetic surgery. There are lessons therein for everyone.

*She got her looks from her father. He was a plastic surgeon.*
— **Groucho Marx**

# 1
# SNAPSHOT of the
# BIG PICTURE

## Considering Cosmetic Surgery?

- Wondering what to expect?

- What you would look like?

- Think you want it but a bit frightened by the prospect?

- Not sure if it is for you because you have not yet researched it?

- Need some help?

- Some concise, to-the-point information?

- Would you like to have an expert, an advisor at your side to coach you and demystify the process of deciding, "*go*" or "*no go*"?

If yes is your answer to all or most of these seven questions, you hold the the guiding light in your hands. ***Let this book be your coach, your personal consultant.*** It can ease the way for you. It will make the decision-making process much easier.

**INSIDER'S INSIGHT**

We can't keep you from getting old, but we can keep you from looking old.

**-RK**

*You do not even have to buy this book to get an overview of the book's content. It is right here, up front, in this first chapter. An easy way to help you decide whether or not to buy the book. No charge; Chapter 1 is on me.*

It will take only ten minutes. If you are at your favorite bookstore, pull up a comfortable chair, grab a cup of coffee, sit and relax a bit. Thumb through this chapter. I am going to give you a sneak preview, a glimpse of what the rest of the chapters will expand upon.

I shall let *you* decide if the book is important for you, if its advice is meaningful, and if you think there is value here. *I'll even share my 16 biggest secrets with you, right now:*

---

## THE 16 MOST IMPORTANT COSMETIC SURGERY SECRETS

**Secret #1.**  Many statisfied cosmetic surgery patients "don't talk." Some of your relations and friends have had something done, but they won't necessarily tell you.

**Secret #2.**  Doctors are flooding into cosmetic surgery. Many lack proper training. Some are incompetent.

**Secret #3.**  Selecting a cosmetic surgeon can be a walk through a minefield. DO YOUR HOMEWORK.

**Secret #4.**  The doctor you want is called a super-specialist—he practices cosmetic surgery *exclusively*.

**Secret #5.**  Many consultations focus on selling, not teaching. When is a "free" consultation too expensive?

**Secret #6.**  A surgeon's "before" and "after" album is filled with clues. You should see lots of photos—and they must be "photographically honest."

**Secret #7.**  Know the 15 smartest questions to ask any cosmetic surgeon.

**Secret #8.**  A consultation without computer imaging has limited value. You need to see, on a computer screen, what you will look like "after."

**Secret #9.**  Fees are negotiable. Know the ropes.

**Secret #10.** The facility in which you have your procedure done can be as important as who is doing it!

> The good physician knows his patients through and through, and his knowledge is bought dearly. Time, sympathy and understanding must be lavishly dispensed, but the reward is to be found in that personal bond which forms the greatest satisfaction of the practice of medicine. One of the essential qualities of the clinician is interest in humanity, for the secret of the care of the patient is in caring for the patient.
>
> **–Francis Weld Peabody, MD, Lecture to Harvard Medical Students, 1927**

**Secret #11.** Combining a trip to an exotic location with cosmetic surgery may be a less-than-perfect mix.

**Secret #12.** Know the difference between an anesthesiologist and an anesthetist. Only one is a medical doctor.

**Secret #13.** High fees don't necessarily mean better results. Low fees are not always a bargain.

**Secret #14.** Your chances of post-surgical complications can be reduced by understanding your doctor's philosophy on "aftercare."

**Secret #15.** Aspirin, herbs, even vitamins can influence your risk during surgery. Be sure to know what to avoid.

**Secret #16.** There is a responsible answer or solution for every concern, worry and reservation.

---

**Yes, I am "giving it away, free."** But that is not an issue for me. What is important is that you get a sense of how very unique and important my insider information is. I am offering to share this with you if you have any interest in improving your appearance.

---

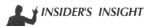 *INSIDER'S INSIGHT*

### *Asking For A Referral?*
### *Here's A Shortcut To The Top Doctors*

When asking a friend, doctor or other source for a referral for cosmetic surgery, be specific. Don't say: "Can you give me the name of a great plastic surgeon?" or "Know a good, reputable cosmetic surgeon?"

That's not specific enough. In today's world of doctors, find a superspecialist— one who is an expert in the procedure you want.

If you are considering changing your nose, the wise "Insider's" question is: "Who's known for great noses?" For body liposuction: "Who has the most experience in liposuction?"

Go straight to a superspecialist.

*-RK*

---

It may be that when you finish reading this chapter, you will have learned enough to conclude that cosmetic surgery is not for you. And that is fine; as good as cosmetic surgery is for those who have it, it is not for everyone. That will be your choice.

In our practice, it is not the right thing for about 20 percent of the patients who consult with me. One of five. I do not want to deflate a patient's dream and often they will describe my respectful decline as "a disappointment." Rather, I am acting professionally by giving them a responsible, realistic, and honest opinion. Doctor and patient must be on the same page and I will help you level the playing field so you can make a decision with confidence. If you are considering cosmetic surgery, selecting your doctor will be one of the most important decisions of your life. And if it is inappropriate for a man or woman to have a procedure, I shall be best serving those who sit in front of me by giving them my best opinion, an answer based on my years of experience, not an answer they would prefer to hear.

> **Most people don't come to a plastic surgeon wanting to look like someone else. Most people still want to look like themselves, but better.**
>
> **-Garry Brody, MD, USC Professor of Clinical Surgery** in *USC Health*, **Spring 2001**

I now tell you what I tell such patients:  I enjoy doing surgery. It is my life's work and obviously, it is the only way I earn my living. But *my first obligation to you is to give my best; not self-serving, opinion. And sometimes, that boils down to one word: "Don't." Don't if your health is not satisfactory. Don't if even a slight risk of a poor outcome or complication is unacceptable. And don't if you are not certain you really want cosmetic surgery.*

That is how I have done it during 25 years of consulting with over ten thousand prospective patients. Skeptics may scoff at hearing of my telling patients—despite their pleadings—that I do not accept the fee and operate if my heart is not in it.  But that is how this doctor practices. It is about integrity—not money—because one, or two, or ten more cases a year will not make a difference in my lifestyle. But, doing surgery without the comfort of knowing that I am doing the right thing would push me over an ethical line I choose not to cross.  I prefer to sleep well.

---

### The Perils of Cosmetic Surgery

*A middle-aged woman is in a terrible accident and is rushed to the hospital. On the way there, her vital signs fail. The doctors are able to revive her, but while she is gone, she sees God and he tells her she has 40 more years to live.*

*Since she is in the hospital, and knowing she is going to be around for a while, she decides to use the stay for self-improvement. She has a facelift, an eyelid lift, and a nose job. She gets released from the hospital and, as she crosses the street, she is run over by a truck and killed.*

*When she sees God again, she says to him, "I thought you said I had 40 years to live"!*

*To which God replies, "I'm sorry…I didn't recognize you."*

---

If you conclude that you want cosmetic surgery, I strongly encourage you to go into this with eyes wide open. *You want to do it right the first time.*

*When performed correctly, cosmetic surgery can transform your life.* However, if you are a deluded optimist, too-trusting, do not use good judgment, or even if your expectations are unreasonable or incorrect, you will be disappointed.

**Fast Face & Body Fact**

**More than 6.3 million women chose to have cosmetic plastic surgery in 2000.**

*-The 2001 Report of the 2000*
*Procedural Statistics,*
**American Society of Plastic Surgeons**

I am going to tell it as it is; the good and the bad and the not-too-pleasant. I'll share some possibilities and potentials, but will also reveal some pitfalls that you never thought about. They are all important. And that is why you will be challenged to do two things: look at yourself in the mirror, and look at the entire subject of cosmetic surgery, because many factors must be considered to give you the insight and result you want.

## This Book Will Answer Your #1 Question: *What Can I Really Expect?*

*Secrets of a Beverly Hills Cosmetic Surgeon* **is written for those of you who want straight talk.** If you will come with me on the journey we are about to begin, I guarantee I will help you decide if cosmetic surgery is right—or not right—for *you.*

Should you decide that either the time is not right or, for whatever personal reason, you are not committed to undergoing surgery, you can learn about popular nonsurgical alternatives. They are not as powerful, but they work: skin care products and in-office medical treatments that are minimally invasive. You will have a taste of how today's cosmetic surgeons and their allies can help you improve your appearance and slow the clock.

This is a mini-encyclopedia of self-improvement. A menu of treatments from light to heavy, from simple office procedures to more elaborate surgical operations. By the last page of the book, you will know what you want—and what you do not want—and hopefully, will thank me for the advice.

## PATIENT COMMENTARY

*This procedure was something I had contemplated for quite a number of years, but I always found a good reason/excuse for not going ahead with it. It was a simple, painless procedure that I had built up in my mind until it became an intimidating prospect involving a huge expense and lots of pain and discomfort. I couldn't have been more wrong. I didn't even take so much as an aspirin while I was recuperating and I was really surprised at how little bruising and swelling was involved. My first thought when I saw my nose after the surgery was "I can't believe I waited all those years!" I still think that when I look in the mirror. I am lucky to have found you when I did, as I can't imagine still walking around with my old nose.*

*So thank you again, Dr. Kotler! You (and my new nose) have made such a positive impact in my life.*

*-Heidi, student*

## The Good, the Bad and the Ugly

For more than a quarter of a century I have been privileged to participate in one of man's more fascinating surgical advances—a gift to himself—the improvement of his appearance. It is an honor to have been chosen by over eight thousand patients to be the doctor who would make a profound and positive change in their lives. In a world where many discretionary purchases and indulgences have a limited lifespan and importance, cosmetic surgery outlasts most, carrying lifelong internal satisfaction.

*In less than one generation cosmetic surgery has become an accepted, mainstream undertaking for millions.* According to the American Society of Plastic Surgeons, "Surgical and nonsurgical cosmetic surgery procedures in the United States increased 31 percent from 1992 to 2000." Americans are expected to have 8 million cosmetic procedures this year. Its expanding popularity reflects these advances:

> **Any good plastic surgeon is and must be a psychologist, whether he would have it so or not. When you change a man's face you almost invariably change his future. Change his physical image and nearly always you change the man—his personality, his behavior—and sometimes even his basic talents and abilities.**
>
> -Maxwell Maltz, MD, FICS, author *Psycho-Cybernetics*

- **Expansion of capability**—new solutions for previously unimprovable conditions.

- **Better results** — natural appearing, not "fake" or artificial.

- **Greater longevity of procedures**—today, there is no reason for a facelift to last only two or three years.

- **Reduction in surgical and anesthesia risks**—through the development of both new equipment and refinement of techniques, risks to patients continue to decrease.

- **Shortened operating times**—this translates to a safer procedure and significantly lower fees, opening the door of opportunity to prospective patients who thought they could not afford cosmetic surgery.

- **Minimized recovery time**—patients can return to work in seven to fourteen days; a decided savings in time and money.

Yet, despite these impressive improvements, poor quality cosmetic surgery still exists. While it is a challenge even for me to spot well-done (natural-appearing) cosmetic surgery, it is easy to spot the "unnatural" work. Whether I am walking down Rodeo Drive in Beverly Hills, Michigan Avenue in Chicago, or Fifth Avenue in New York or even Illinois Avenue in Green Lake, Wisconsin, I have noticed the overdone, too-scooped, too-short, nostrils-flaring nose job; or the over-tightened, over-pulled, walking-through-a-wind-tunnel facelift. Instinctively, I wince. I'm sorry an opportunity for success was missed. In the right hands, our specialty can do better—and does so every day.

## A MOTHER'S COMMENTARY

> *I feel so badly concerning the results of my daughter's nose surgery. It was done by the Chairman of the Department at one of the local medical schools. Only afterward did I find out that most of his time was spent doing reconstructive surgery, not cosmetic surgery, and that particularly he had very little experience doing nasal surgery. My assumption that the Department Chairman at a university was the best person to do the procedure was very poor.*
>
> *–Mother of teenage patient at consultation for correction of a poorly performed nasal surgery*

People are often frightened away from cosmetic surgery as a result of these botched jobs. Unfortunately, some prospective patients have deferred consulting about a cosmetic procedure because of rumors, or first-hand accounts shared by friends or family members of (avoidable) pain and suffering.

These negatives raise a question: *is there a common factor responsible for (a) poor results that some people sustain, (b) the inappropriate, unfounded fears and skepticism that prevent others from achieving their wish for an improvement in appearance? What is wrong? What is the problem?*

*The answer, the diagnosis, is lack of adequate, correct information.* More and better information is needed: ideally insider information—from an expert, from a source working daily in the trenches of the specialty. Sound advice, parallel to what I seek when choosing professionals for my family or myself. I do not know very much about the inner workings of the architectural, accounting or legal professions. But 35 years after receiving my medical degree, I do know about my profession. Some cosmetic surgery books chronicle individual patient experiences, and others delve deeply into the technical aspects and minutiae of every major and minor procedure. No book, however, has ever revealed the inner workings of this specialty. The culture, the politics, the interspecialty rivalries. And the biggest problem: *the wrong surgeons doing cosmetic surgery.*

> **According to the licensing laws of most states, any licensed physician, regardless of training and experience, may declare himself a plastic surgeon. For that matter, any licensed physician may limit his practice and declare himself a practitioner of any specialty he may select.**
>
> **-Kurt J. Wagner, MD and Gerald Imber, MD,** authors, *Beauty by Design*

This is the first behind-the-scenes peek at American cosmetic surgery from one of its own, a bona fide insider, not a professional writer on assignment. An authoritative exposé of this much-discussed—but poorly understood—specialty. A primer on how you can safely navigate through what is the best way for you to obtain the best possible results.

In cosmetic surgery, there should be only excellence. After all, this specialty is about results, and the results are seen by all. I believe the percentage of unhappy experiences is too high, despite the availability of enough sophisticated practitioners. The glitz, glamour, and inane celebrity-slanted TV and magazine stories have displaced the meaningful, dispassionate advice needed to make a wise consumer decision. While cosmetic surgery is not a frequent undertaking, it cries out for the same thoughtful, objective analysis as any major purchase. You want to do it well; a poor result cannot necessarily be corrected.

## PATIENT COMMENTARY

> *I consulted with the doctor who said he 'did not really like doing nasal surgery, but would do it for me.' Why would I ever want him to 'do it for me' if he was not happy doing it?*
>
> *-Carole, businesswoman, California*

Since cosmetic surgery is always elective, you have the luxury of time. Time to do the research, the study, the investigation, so you do it right the first time. What I am telling you is that such a search is not quick, nor simple. You are going to have to dig a bit. You are going to

**The general stigma surrounding cosmetic plastic surgery as something done only by the vain and rich is vanishing.**

**-Walter Erhardt, MD American Society of Plastic Surgeons**

have to work. Once again, that old maxim that your parents told you applies: "You get out of something what you put into it." While it is quick and effortless to open your *Yellow Pages* and call the first doctor with the most eye-grabbing ad, I submit that you will not be doing yourself a favor, but rather a bit of dice-rolling. Are long shot odds acceptable to you? If so, I suggest the racetrack. Otherwise, read on.

Mine is a rather unique specialty and an uncommon business. Consider this: Cosmetic surgery is a distinct medical specialty, provided by physicians but, unlike all other specialties, cosmetic surgery does not treat illness. Cosmetic surgeons often have more professional interaction with hair stylists and makeup artists than they do with other physicians.

Cosmetic surgery is a learned profession, but operates more like a business, prospering through marketing, advertising and price competition. But the fees are inconsistent. For the buyer trying to correlate price with the usual variables of quality and service, the

**81 percent of 680 workers surveyed by the American Academy of Facial Plastic and Reconstructive Surgery say they would tell co-workers they have had a nose job; only 71 percent would tell friends.**

*Wall Street Journal,* **December 5 2001**

search is perplexing indeed. Further complicating doctor selection is that today's cosmetic surgeons —from varying educational and training backgrounds, and different specialties—purport to deliver the same services. This is "specialty overlap," and it is explained in **Chapter 3, Selecting the Right Surgeon.** This competition between specialties for the same work makes it harder to select a cosmetic surgeon than it is to choose an electrician. And, this confusion is worsening for you, the consumer. More and more doctors—disheartened and demoralized by the depersonalization of managed care served up by uncaring, profit-driven insurance companies—are now moving into cosmetic surgery. This doctor flight is a big concern to those of us in medical education.

*Cosmetic surgery, wrapped in hope and packaged with excitement, is too often unwisely driven by emotion.* The prospective patient can be confused by media coverage that can be poorly researched and sensation-oriented. The checkout line at your grocery store is littered with the latest, enticing celebrity exposés. But there is no meaningful information for those eager to gather solid facts about the specialty.

Ironically, the people who can best help you understand this road less traveled are those who have had cosmetic surgery. However, many patients do not disclose their surgery. Your co-worker returning from vacation looking "rested" may give credit to a "sleepy little spot" she found rather than the surgeon she visited. How can you get an education when the voices of experience are silent?

> **At one point, I was called the Queen of Plastic Surgery. I did bring it out of the closet. After I talked about all my tucks and jobs, people opened up about theirs. I would be sitting on the couch on the Tonight Show, and someone would lean over and say, "I just had my eyes done" or whatever. I became the clearinghouse for everyone, because I knew all the answers. The surgeons loved me. I loved demystifying.**
>
> **-Phyllis Diller quoted in *Time*, June 2001**

The bottom line is that the consumer has nowhere to go. The media talks too much drivel, the veterans may not talk at all and specialty overlap is confusing. This realization inspired me to share the information I have gathered over 35 years as a physician about what some people still consider a "closet" subject. Who better to tell it to you like it is?

This insight is why this book is my personal mission. I see no reason to keep any of this information secret— cosmetic surgery is too good and too important, but only when done properly. *I want to help you avoid the unfortunate result—whether it be overdone, underdone, or burdened with complications.* Although you need not learn the surgical technicalities of taking a bump off the nose or sculpting the neck or removing a wrinkle, you can learn the formula for finding the most qualified professionals who will do the best possible job for you.

**INSIDER'S INSIGHT**

Too soon we grow old, too late we grow smart.
-Adage
This book is the antidote to both contentions.
-RK

With this book my objectives are:

● **To present important informatio**n—known within our specialty—and unknown to the public.

● **To outline a clear, rational methodology** by which you can research cosmetic surgery and choose the best doctor to serve you.

● **To provide you an easy-to-follow manual** and specific tools (smart questions) with which to conduct your search.

My experience as a surgeon began as a resident trainee in 1968. The length and depth of my personal history as a physician qualifies me to help you better understand the inner workings of today's cosmetic surgery because the world of medicine is different from what existed when I opened my practice. You need to learn—within the context of the rapid changes that have visited the medical profession—how this new health care climate has created a fresh set of challenges for physicians. **Managed Care has driven many doctors to retool and begin doing cosmetic surgery.** But that migration often translates to inconsistent patient results given the absence of formalized and adequate training—under expert supervision—heretofore the hallmark of medical education. Yes, it may say "Plastic Surgery" or "Cosmetic Surgery" on the office door, but you must find out more about the kind of plastic or cosmetic surgery the doctor performs, and his qualifications to do it.

> I don't know how things are in California today, but in Florida, they are awful. We have family practitioners and ophthalmologists doing full body liposuction, anesthesiologists doing breast augmentation and oral surgeons, dermatologists and ophthalmologists doing face lifts—all quite legally! It seems everyone wants to be a plastic surgeon. I can understand since it is a wonderful and very gratifying profession…and the "cash on the barrelhead" nature of cosmetic surgery is certainly attractive in this day of declining reimbursement from third-party insurers. What I cannot understand is the pell-mell rush to discard our long-established residency training system in order to allow a few individuals to circumvent the formal training process and call themselves plastic surgeons.
>
> **-Richard T. Bosshardt, MD, FACS**
> *Bulletin of the American College of Surgeons,* **May 2001**

Choosing an amateur or rookie without the right resume is a recipe for failure. Your road to a safe, comfortable experience and "great result" will take you on a specialist recognition course. You will learn how to pick the most appropriate and highly skilled doctor.

Of all your decisions, this is the most critical. Stumble here and you are down the wrong road. You will learn about superspecialists—the specialist's specialist, if you will. Doctors at the pinnacle of training, experience, focus and performance. The superstars of the medical profession.

To find these superstars, you will have to do some sifting and winnowing. But I shall make it smoother and easier for you. In **Chapter 3, Selecting the Right Surgeon,** you will learn how to eliminate second-string players by one short call to an office or a quick peek at a professional biography. That way, you won't waste precious time and your hard-earned dollars in a consultation with the wrong doctor.

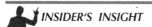 *INSIDER'S INSIGHT*

### <u>Superspecialist For Your Auto But Not For Yourself?</u>

Consider the importance of focus and specialization, think about that certified car mechanic who works only on your imported car, for example. Given a choice between the corner gas station repairman who claims to "fix everything," and the factory trained technician, who will be likely to fix your car the first time? Today's automobiles have an average of 15,000 moving parts. Is it possible for any mechanic to become an expert in the inner workings of dozens of car models? Doesn't **your** human body—the only one you'll ever own—deserve the most specialized repairman?

*-RK*

*You sort and select by knowing the smart questions to ask at each level of research,* up to and through the consultation. Treat the consultation as an interview. While the surgeon is evaluating you medically, you are evaluating him for an appropriate match. Study this book well, my friend, and you will earn an A+ in Cosmetic Surgery Consultation. And, you should fight for that A+ because this is so important to you. You want no regrets, no remorse, no whining that you did not do enough homework. You want the best possible result. Because when your cosmetic surgery result is good, a big, wide smile looks back at you from your mirror.

## Look Closely at That *Before and After* Album

Once you are savvy enough to consult with superspecialists (the ones who perform cosmetic surgery exclusively), how do you then choose among this already select talent pool? You begin by critically examining before and after photos. You must look at them as analytically as an auction house examines a work of art. I will coach you and teach you visual analysis. You will know how to use the practice's "before and after" albums as a measurement of what you are buying: the doctor's talent as displayed in his art form.

## Why Not See What You'll Look Like?

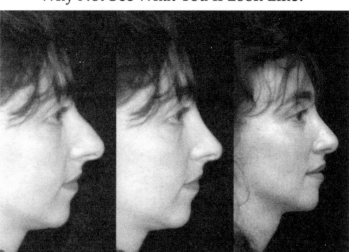

*Computer imaging, three views. (1) Left: "before." (2) Middle: "computer imaged preview." (3) Right: "final result: nasal surgery and chin augmentation."*

Top quality, informative, valuable consultations must include a computer-generated transformation of your "before" photo into a satisfactory "after." Otherwise, it is all guesswork. Who buys something without seeing it? You don't want to sign up for nasal surgery, facelift, or breast augmentation without knowing what you will look like after the surgery. Today's remarkable computer technology can show you a preview, a realistic prediction of the new you. It answers that lurking question: "What will I look like...after?" And a conscientious cosmetic surgeon tries to obtain even better results.

> If you've been tempted to try cosmetic surgery but have always held back, what I've described may have piqued your interest sufficiently so that you're ready to cross the threshold. In that case, you'll want to devote a good deal of time and energy to choosing the right surgeon. I've had some experience with all this, and I know how important it is to make that choice, yet how difficult it can sometimes be to choose wisely.
>
> -Kathy Keeton, author
> *Longevity: The Science of Staying Young*

## Some Operating Rooms Are Safer than Others

Would you like to know if the facility meets demanding safety standards? If it has a medical *"Good Housekeeping® Seal of Approval"*? Every day you enter buildings that require an occupancy-safety license to

* The above patient after seeing the computer image of the predicted result, opted, just before surgery, to improve her profile by adding the chin augmentation.

keep the doors open. You then ride up and down in elevators that are regularly inspected and licensed. You cannot operate a potentially dangerous 4,000-pound machine—called an automobile—without an operator's license.

Doesn't it make sense that a facility where you are deliberately rendered unconscious—and therefore helpless—be credentialed and meet strict code standards for structural integrity, fire protection and even earthquake resistance? Big risks will be avoided by knowing the difference between an unlicensed, unaccredited, never-inspected facility, large or small, and a state-licensed, U.S. government-certified, independently accredited, specialized outpatient surgery center, or a fully accredited hospital. There are accepted guidelines for evaluating surgical facilities. You must know about them.

## Don't Forget to Ask About Anesthesia

While most people focus on the cosmetic surgery itself, they fail to realize that the big risk is not the "cutting and sewing"—it is the anesthetic. That is why I shall teach you the difference between professionals who aid the surgeon by administering the anesthetic. *Do you know the difference between an anesthetist and an anesthesiologist?* The former are nurses, the latter are physician-specialists. Think about who will be at the controls during your surgery.

## Insider Information Is Precious
## When You Discuss Dollars

I shall level the playing field and arm you with negotiation strategies that will save you money. Here is a sample: understanding that it makes good business sense for a doctor to operate on two or more patients (not at the same time, of course), at a reduced "group rate" can translate into significant savings for you and a surgery partner. The efficiency of this practice converts to a discounted fee; more on this in **Chapter 6, "About Fees" and Chapter 10, "Erasing Mental Blocks."**

Having your procedure on a "stand by" basis or opting for prepayment can also help lower your cost. Since the individual cash outlay can be $5,000 to $10,000, a saving of 15 to 20 percent equals hundreds or thousands of dollars. Good business for your doctor can be great savings for you. Do you wonder how cosmetic surgeons price their services? And, one of the secrets that may surprise you, is that the *most skilled superspecialists are not necessarily the most expensive.* **Chapter 6** reveals the explanation.

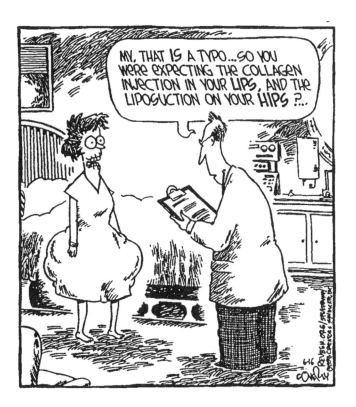

## You Don't Want the Ball to Be Dropped
## Before or After Surgery

The practice you want will give you old-fashioned, one-on-one, attentive care. Top practices prepare you for everything and anticipate your needs.

**The best cosmetic surgery practices provide for your total care from beginning to end:**

- *Make sure you are fit for surgery*— healthy.

- *Give you written instructions* telling you what to expect, before and after, and answer all questions.

- *Provide routine medications and supplies.* Your needs are anticipated.

- *Make house calls, if necessary.*   (Yes, you read that correctly).

While cosmetic surgeons do not cure cancer, give you a new liver, or replace a worn-out hip, we are still medical doctors, not—as some would paint us—highly-educated beauticians. Many of us still know how to give that now-elusive patient care. The best practices give it. These are the practices you should seek. I can show you the way.

If you have relatives or friends in the cosmetic surgery world, you are fortunate because you automatically have insider information. They will lead you down the right path. But if you do not have a brother, cousin or best friend who is a cosmetic surgeon, you are still in luck; I shall fill the pathfinder role for you. The knowledge you are about to gain is important; cosmetic surgery—despite the hype—is not trivial. It is not casual surgery. It is about your body. There is a bit more complexity to cosmetic surgery than you thought. You must be vigilant. Forewarned is forearmed.

The most important secret from this Beverly Hills cosmetic surgeon is that there are too many secrets about cosmetic surgery. Too much hype, too many silly, shallow celebrity stories, and too little practical, important, even life-saving information.

Appearance is a subjective and emotionally charged subject. However, changing your appearance surgically should never be based solely on emotion. Instead, there is a prescribed methodology to selecting a proper surgeon, opting for the appropriate procedure, and choosing a comfortable, safe location.

My hope is that this book will influence your approach by erasing myths, misconceptions, and misrepresentations, making your research process unintimidating, efficient, and satisfying. I want you to enjoy the best possible result reflected in your mirror.

# Dental panel targets cometic surgery

**HEALTH:** The illegal practice by oral surgeons has been ignored but now faces probable penalties.

**By KIMBERLY KINDY**
The Orange County Register

Oral surgeons performing illegal facial cosmetic surgery in California will likely be punished with large fines, jail time, permanent marks on their records — even the loss of their dental licenses.

The state Dental Board of Examiners is expected Friday to approve a list of proposed crackdowns.

"We are sending a very strong message," said Dr. Peter Hartman, a general dentist and dental board member. "I don't think anyone who is performing these procedures should be confused about where we stand on the issue and what might happen."

Oral and maxillofacial surgeons typically hold dental but not medical licenses. Some

also have medical degrees, meaning they can perform the procedures.

The procedures in question are those that venture too far from the jaw and mouth and aren't related to dentistry.

For years, the dental board has looked the other way as some oral surgeons performed eyelid surgery, neck liposuction, even face lifts. It has investigated only when something went wrong and someone complained.

The board went after the oral surgeons — who frequent-

ly advertise their illegal work — after a series of stories in The Orange County Register revealed that the practice is widespread.

"Until now, there was no real incentive for them to change their behavior," said state Sen. Liz Figueroa, D-Fremont, who chairs a committee that oversees the dental board. "This puts them on notice. People are watching now, and there are consequences."

▶ **BOARD:** Oral surgeons to be put on notice. **News 14**

*Orange County, CA newspaper reveals crackdown on dental specialists performing facial cosmetic surgery. January 8, 2000.*
*(Notice their typo in headline.)*

The next chapter—which may be a bit of a shocker—is titled, **"The Terrible Truth About Some Cosmetic Surgeons."** But, better to know sooner than later, before rather than after.

## Why Do Some Celebrities Look So Bad After Cosmetic Surgery?

That's a question often asked by prospective patients. The common assumption is that money, power and access should automatically guarantee garnering top cosmetic surgery talent. Not always.

I see three reasons why some celebrities look so bad after cosmetic surgery. Bad luck is not one of them.

1. **Bad decision making.** Celebrities—like the rest of us—are not immune from making bad purchasing decisions. They are not anointed with special wisdom because of their fame. They may not do enough research to sort out the most talented practitioners for their particular needs. Or they rely on a manager or advisor to conduct the search. Off the screen, away from the studio, they own no magic, no divining rod to lead them to the right offices. They need to do their homework; just like you.

2. **Not knowing when to stop.** When you see obvious and overdone cosmetic surgery on the face of a celebrity, it usually announces that they did not know when to stop. They kept going beyond reason. Perhaps the celebs were unwisely shooting for perfection, for immortality. But they are on a hopeless chase. Regardless of who is famous or otherwise, the same rules of life govern us all.

3. **A cosmetic surgeon who falls into the celebrity trap**. He, too, drops common sense. He forgets that mantra his mentors hammered into his memory bank: *"The pursuit of perfection is the ultimate enemy of good."* Overdoing is always worse than underdoing. That it is easier to add on later, but almost impossible to "put back that which you took off." But why does an ordinarily objective and wise doctor temporarily discard the sound advice his teachers gave him? Because, he, too, has a chance to be a celebrity, however vicarious. An opportunity to bask in that special glow we Americans are so good at fostering is often too hard to pass up.

Media personalities are attractive, smart and charming; that is how they reached their level of success and fame. They can be very manipulative, very convincing in their arguments. Isn't that their craft? That is why, it is hard to say "no" to the lady or gentleman sitting in front of you whose face may be recognized by billions of people. And, perhaps subconsciously, the doctor wants to say yes, wants to satisfy this important person, to ingratiate himself, to join the club, to be part of that special world. It can be heady stuff.

Consulting with famous people is very difficult. I have been there many times. The doctor must harness his best instincts, his purest motives, his strongest common sense to do the right thing for every patient regardless of status. Not for himself, his ego, his office's "wall of fame" photo display, or his bank account.

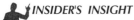 **INSIDER'S INSIGHT**

### A Celebrity's Cosmetic Surgery Disaster

Years ago comedian Totie Fields died because of a cosmetic misadventure. Knowing that Totie was obese and diabetic should have been a bright enough red flag for any conscientious cosmetic surgeon to decline to operate.

Totie developed a blocked artery which led to to her complications, snowballing to her tragic premature death.

I share this to remind you that the first decision about cosmetic surgery is whether or not it is right to do it. In the "reasons not to do it" column, at the top, always stands: "Medical condition(s); too risky."

I urge you to consult with a doctor whose practice is not a cosmetic surgery conveyer belt. You want a doctor who thinks first and operates second.

*-RK*